THE COURAGE TO CARE

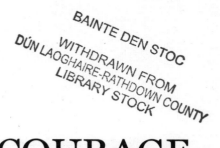
THE COURAGE TO CARE

A Call for Compassion

Christie Watson

Chatto & Windus

LONDON

1 3 5 7 9 10 8 6 4 2

Chatto & Windus, an imprint of Vintage,
20 Vauxhall Bridge Road,
London SW1V 2SA

Chatto & Windus is part of the Penguin Random House
group of companies whose addresses can be found at
global.penguinrandomhouse.com

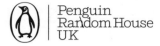

Penguin
Random House
UK

First published by Chatto & Windus in 2020

penguin.co.uk/vintage

A CIP catalogue record for this book is available from
the British Library

ISBN 9781784742980

Noam Chomsky is quoted from *Language and Mind*
(New York: Harcourt Brace Jovanovich, 1972), p. 112

Typeset in 10/18 pt Miller Text
Integra Software Services Pvt. Ltd, Pondicherry

Printed and bound in Great Britain by Clays Ltd, Elcograf S.p.A.

Penguin Random House is committed to a sustainable future
for our business, our readers and our planet. This book is
made from Forest Stewardship Council® certified paper.

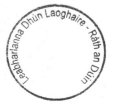
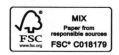

For the Families of Nurses

I know you're tired, but come. This is the way.

Rumi

Contents

Author's Note

The events described here are based on memories of my experiences as a nurse. Identifying features have been changed in order to protect the privacy of colleagues, patients and their families, and descriptions of certain individuals and situations have been merged to further protect identities. Any similarities are purely coincidental.

Introduction

The Language of Kindness, my previous book, focused on my experiences, primarily as a hospital nurse, in uniform. But there is a whole world of nursing outside hospitals, spanning the length and breadth of our country, and countless nurses' voices which deserve to be heard. I spent two years writing *The Courage to Care* and was lucky enough to travel widely, meeting nurses from all walks of life, and hearing about their incredible work. I wanted to write about exceptional nurses everywhere, in every setting, and the difference they make to the lives of colleagues, patients and families, including my own.

I have been talking and writing about the importance of nurses for many years: how undervalued they have been; how overworked and underpaid; and underlining just how vital nurses are to society. But of course, I had no idea what was to come. None of us did. I was making final edits to *The Courage to Care* when COVID-19 changed the world, perhaps forever.

This is a time of profound reflection for all of us. We must pause and mourn, and grieve for those who have died during this awful virus. Perhaps we can continue to honour them – and all those frontline workers who lost their lives for us – by taking care of our neighbours, our communities, and the vulnerable, including those who are unable to work and those who are no longer working. Those in need. People have been thinking of other families, as well as their own. We must hold onto that: the courage to care. Compassion for others is how we will be judged. And it is how we should be judged. This is a time for all of us to think about community, how delicate life is, and what life now means. We will be changed by this, all of us. And the search for meaning has only just begun.

I had no idea how poignant and timely this book would be. Nurses have always been at the forefront of society, and that, perhaps, is finally being acknowledged. It is nurses who are saving lives during all of this, and the lack of critical care nurses has been one of the most significant challenges. It is nurses who are holding the hands of our loved ones as they are dying, who are with them when we can't be there, reminding us that we are never alone, not even now. And it will be nurses who bear the weight of COVID-19 long after the peak. Because, for those who survive, this is just the beginning. The level of support, rehab and expert care needed by so many people is almost unimaginable, and the fallout for those who have suffered – due to the impact of COVID-19 – with other illnesses and diseases is beyond measure. Those with cancer, long-term conditions, mental illness. An entire generation of children. Our elderly. Nurses have always fought for social justice and human rights, and COVID-19 has shown up the vast inequalities and discrimination across our country. It will be those who already suffer most who will suffer more, and nurses will care for and champion them, regardless.

Yet nurses – predominantly women – remain undervalued even now.

The absence of any nurse on the COVID-19 SAGE advisory panel, for example, is – or should be, surely – unacceptable to all of us. The reason, I am told, is that SAGE is made up of scientists.

But, of course, nurses *are* scientists. And writers. And academics and philosophers and leaders and researchers and artists and experts and technicians and practitioners and innovators and entrepreneurs and influencers and statisticians and workforce modellers and expert witnesses and advanced practitioners and crisis managers. Nurses are consistently cited by the public as the most trusted profession.

It is high time that nurses of every background have a seat at the political table – for all our sakes. Nurses have never been more important.

6 July 2020

1

A Shrinking Satsuma

My daughter. She is here. Curled up in a hedgehog ball, but softer than anything in the universe. Not wanting to miss a blink's worth of time, I gaze at her face, her pouting mouth, the way she frowns, yawns. Her shell-ears. She is born with a quiff of thick black hair and an expression that says she's been here before. A knowing, testing look. Her eyes are such dark brown that it is only when I tilt her into the pale light from the window slats, letting it stripe across her face, that I see they are not black. Her skin is shockingly white, but the maternity support worker, Mary, laughs and holds up my daughter's tiny hands, shows me her fingernails. 'She will soon change' she says. 'Look.' And her nailbeds are dark, the colour I expected her to be, with a black dad, white mum.

That she is born whiter than I am is not my only shock. She has a large Mongolian spot on the base of her spine, a congenital dermal melanocytosis, a type of birthmark. It is purple-grey, the colour of an old bruise and the size of a satsuma. She is early, and small. The midwife tells me it's nothing to worry about, but worry is born when she is. I've read research that suggests Mongolian spots are not, as previously thought, always benign. They can be associated with metabolic disorders, and with other diseases and conditions. I try to explain this fear that I feel in my stomach and throat and hair to the midwife, the cleaner and, finally, to Mary, who brings me lukewarm sweet tea and two gingernut biscuits. But it's hard to put into words. Maybe she is seriously ill? Perhaps I am being irrational? I begin assessing my baby as if she's one of my intensive-care patients. I check her reflexes, pupil reaction, respiratory rate and capillary-refill time.

Mary watches me assessing her and laughs. 'Nurses and doctors – always the worst patients.' She scoops up my daughter in one hand and holds her face close. 'She's hungry.' Right on cue, my daughter makes a gulping, sucking sound, and squawks and squawks. Mary helps me attach her to my breast and it feels like fire as she feeds, burning through my centre: a needle-sharp pain, totally unfamiliar. Mary tells me it is normal. 'You get used to it, that sensation. And then you miss it when it's gone. My daughter has a daughter of her own now.'

I look down. The idea is impossible. She will be a baby for ever, of course. She begins to cough, to splutter and choke, and I hold her upright with shaking hands, imagining milk in her lungs, leading to aspirational pneumonia, ventilation and chronic lung disease. These are my split-second thoughts. How quickly they travel, how dark they become. I didn't think I would be like this. Surely motherhood will be easy for me as a paediatric nurse?

I work as a clinical educator and senior sister in a London Paediatric Intensive Care Unit (PICU). I'm used to high-pressured environments, limited sleep, a stressful life. I work twelve-and-a-half-hour shifts and travel three hours on top of that. My daughter's dad is a hospital consultant, also in intensive care. Our daily life is one of emergencies – the sickest patients you could think of – no sleep and managing stress. I had imagined maternity leave would be a bit of a break. How relaxed I will be, I thought, how Zen. My understanding that most childhood ailments are mild viruses or head colds means I'll be able to spot anything more serious, so I won't need to sweat the small stuff.

Now, though, I am not worried. I'm hysterical.

I list to myself respiratory illnesses that my daughter might catch, and the types of bacteria, fungi and viruses prevalent in winter. What if she contracts a bacterial infection that is resistant to antibiotics? Or a new virus that we can't yet treat? What if she rolls over in her sleep and suffocates? What if my earring falls out into her cot and she chokes on it? *What if, what if, what if …*

I try not to think of all the babies, children and adults I have ever cared for who were seriously ill, but I can't stop. I pace the ward with my newborn, a comma on my shoulder, pressing my teeth together so hard that I can hear cracking noises in my mouth, and I try and push away thoughts of medical conditions, accidents or illnesses. They rush back at me, stinging in succession: congenital heart defects; sepsis; metabolic abnormality; cystic fibrosis; ureteropelvic junction obstruction; liver disease; intussusception; meningitis; RSV; tracheoesophageal fistula; hydrocephalus; neurogenic bladder. That she is jaundiced but otherwise completely healthy does not comfort me; cardiac conditions declare themselves around seven days, when the patent duct in the heart closes and an otherwise healthy baby becomes blue around the edges and dangerously ill, while sepsis can cause a baby or child to become life-threateningly sick within hours. Sometimes minutes.

Memories light up inside me: a child who choked on a piece of bread at nursery, sustaining a hypoxic ischaemic brain injury so severe that he never woke up again; another who drowned in a bath; a baby who fell out of a window; a toddler electrocuted; twins burned by a pulled-over kettle; children with sickle cell disease screaming in pain; a baby girl not much older than mine, crushed by a falling fridge. My head fills with patients who have acute respiratory distress syndrome, or have been run over, kicked by horses, bitten by dogs; patients who are riddled with worms, or lice, or superbugs, or cancer. Babies and children falling from trees or down holes, or hanging from blind cords or cutting themselves to ribbons. Those who drink antifreeze or swallow iron tablets, or antidepressants and end up with damaged hearts, or throats, or kidneys. All of them flash before me as I hold my daughter in the maternity room.

Firefly memories of all the patients I've ever looked after flicker between us. It is utterly terrifying.

She is only hours old, not quite real yet, almost translucent and cobwebbed in blue veins, her arms and legs twitching, coming to life, almost as if she is dancing with my ghosts. I track her movements, scanning for abnormality. Perhaps this is PTSD (post-traumatic stress disorder), repressed for my entire career, but finally expressed after this overwhelming rush of hormones? I need to think rationally. To appreciate this first day of her life, and of my life as a mother. I am born too today, in a way. There is nothing to worry about. We are lucky. I breathe. And breathe. *Breathe.*

But even when breathing, my head travels to people who are not.

Mary pops back in, carrying a jug of water and a cardboard cup. She sees my tears, the shock, the worry; she's seen hyper-anxiety before. 'Childbirth is a soul breaking in two,' she says. 'When she cries, you will feel it in your bones. That's how it is. How it always is.'

I realise that when my daughter hurts, I will hurt more. For ever. And she is not hurting. She is fine. But something in me shifts. I think of the faces of the mothers and fathers and aunts and uncles and grandparents of my patients through all my years of paediatric nursing. I try and imagine their primal pain. How could I not have appreciated the extent of it? I think of friends and family who have had sick children,

5

and children affected by a life-changing diagnosis or accident. In the most desperate of unimaginable horrors, in the face of disability, or serious illness, or pain, or loss, how do patients' families stand upright? How do they find the courage to care?

How could I imagine a love like this?

I can't stop thinking about mothers. The hundreds of mothers I've worked with, the pain they suffered and somehow endured. Their bravery. I think of my own mum and of the things she's endured.

I pull my daughter closer and kiss her. She smells of honeysuckle, and salt, of Plasticine when the packet is first opened, and warm bread, and blood. She is perfect. I feel like a fraud to worry so much. Later I will rationalise it as some sort of survivor's guilt. It is not a common job that I have, and it has warped my sense of reality. Friends who are medical tell me that having children when you know too much goes one way or another: either extreme anxiety or total, horizontally relaxed parenting. In time, I will change from one thing to the other. My children will beg me to let them visit the GP, as if the surgery is a mythical land filled with unicorns. They will never have a day off school, and they will never be sick. Not really. Because I know what sick looks like.

But for now I am swallowed by the feeling that someone has ripped out my heart and laid it on my chest, and I watch her – my beating, bloody heart – and I am consumed. I will do my best to be a good enough mum, I whisper. I'll do my best to be a good enough daughter. I'll try as hard as I can. I'll try and remember what other mothers have taught me. What I have learned from so many families. I kiss my daughter on the forehead, breathe in her smell and tell her how lucky we are, how grateful I am, how blessed. I'll try not to worry. I'll never take this for granted, I promise her, and I promise myself. *Remember, remember, remember.*

Like nature, health and illness have seasons, and nursing varies, depending on the time of year. January is the busiest month by far. Hospitals every year have winter crises that come as a logistical shock, no matter how carefully they are planned for. Bacteria and viruses thrive in the cold. Flu epidemics, bronchiolitis, pneumonia and norovirus are great lovers of January – always a new strain or a mutation, something we didn't foresee or that is difficult to treat – as if nature is reminding us somehow that we are small. People's immunity is generally diminished, while the elderly are vulnerable to winter, to poverty and biting cold. For those who can afford it, central heating and plenty of socialising over the Christmas period render people susceptible, meaning that those with long-term and underlying conditions, such as heart disease, cancer or autoimmune conditions, can get very sick, very quickly. Babies born prematurely the previous year bounce back to the hospital to be ventilated again, their lungs weak from the mechanical ventilation the first time around and vulnerable to winter infections. We see some children every year, sometimes caring for them until adulthood.

Then there are those who are vulnerable to illnesses in January because their immune system is damaged or, in some rare cases, almost non-existent. Patients like Shona, who can't fight infection at all. It is the late 1990s and the infectious-diseases ward at the children's hospital where I am a student nurse is filled with children with a diagnosis of HIV or AIDS, and Shona is one of them. These are the days when AIDS is life-limiting and, often, a death sentence. I have lost two friends already to the virus – one of them a nurse. We are all trying to make sense of this devastating illness, to provide some hope or comfort for the families we're caring for. But we are many years yet from hope. This is a pandemic, although we don't yet understand what that means.

Empress, Shona's mum, has her feet in two countries, Kenya and England – a shadow spreading widely across maps. She was a teacher in a school of 2,000 students, where the children worked hard, achieved well and listened carefully to her quiet but strong voice. But when her daughter became sick, Empress had to give up her job, spending weeks and sometimes months in the hospital, sleeping on a camp bed next to Shona, holding her hand tightly, even in sleep. 'It is wicked,' Empress tells me. 'A cruel and wicked thing.' And then, 'Look at Shona's face. How beautiful she is when she is dreaming.'

I listen in the near-darkness as I slowly administer medication into a vein in Shona's thin arm, the smell of antiseptic stinging the air. I take my time and give the drug more slowly than usual: Empress talks less when I'm doing less, I've noticed, and more when I'm engaged in a task. I am new to nursing, but already I understand that the relationship I build with Empress is as important as the drug I am giving her daughter. Maybe more so. And thankfully, with only three children to care for this evening, I have time to care properly. The nature of the ward and the patients means that although the children are often very sick, they are mostly stable or, if deteriorating, they are doing so slowly. We have three staff nurses and one other student on duty tonight, and it's quiet enough that we can plan sleep breaks. Like most nurses, we sleep a bit whenever we can on night shifts – sometimes for an hour, very occasionally for more, taking it in turns.

Nurses on night shifts who manage to fit in at least a bit of sleep always, always, make the ward more safe, in my experience, never less. A short sleep results in clearer thinking, and the nights I've worked with no sleep whatsoever – which are many – I've felt fuzzy and nowhere near sharp enough to do the job properly. And I'm not alone. More than half of all trainee hospital doctors have had an accident or near-miss on their way home after a night shift, due to sleep deprivation. Hospitals are beginning to introduce sleep pods for staff on night duty, which can only be a good thing. I have missed many a train stop the morning after a night shift when it was too busy for any rest at work, waking up an hour later in the middle of nowhere, with another two-hour journey to get home. Some mornings, if I'm particularly tired, I go home with a handwritten sign on my chest scribbled onto a paper hand towel: *Please wake me up at Brockley*. Someone always gently shakes me awake at the right station.

Empress eventually falls asleep in a gap between disturbances: the observations and medications that slice through her own and Shona's nights. I sit at the nurses' station eating the chicken adobo that one of my nurse friends has brought in (she always comes with home-cooked food to share with her colleagues). There is a pile of trashy magazines and some cups of coffee on the desk and it's quiet, except for the hum of the giant fridge in the medication room next door. I am ignoring the magazines and am instead reading about Acheron, the river of sorrow, described by Virgil as the darkest river of all, yet in the *Suda* as a place of light. Hospitals too are full of light and dark, and nursing involves understanding that dark and light do not necessarily match up with life and death. We are all things at once. I find as much information about nursing in the Greek classics as in *How to Understand and Interpret an ECG Made Simple*. Reading the classics reminds me how little we understand about life and death and the universe, whether we are philosophers or poets or theologists or doctors or scientists, or even nurses. Life doesn't give any answers; only more questions. But literature helps me find meaning in those questions. And I don't know it yet, but a year later I will fail my final nursing exam and will have to pick up *How to Understand and Interpret an ECG Made Simple* after all. Twenty-five years after that, I'll be reaching for my textbooks once more, and this time in a rush.

Empress seems to have answers to some of the difficult questions, though. 'Faith is not knowing. It's hoping,' she tells me. She has a way of explaining that simply makes sense. She laughs. 'Unless you can explain things to a child in a way they understand, then you don't really understand yourself.'

I am nineteen – not a child, but not far off. The nurse–patient relationship is a strange power balance, and it feels odd caring for people who know so much more about life than I do. Empress is older, wiser and more experienced, and she has dedicated her life since the diagnosis to getting Shona the help she needs. But that hasn't been enough. Due to her failed immune system, Shona has developed pneumocystis pneumonia, a serious lung infection, and has since been diagnosed with full-blown AIDS, rather than HIV; this nasty pneumonia and respiratory illness in the immunosuppressed is a battle of mucus and blueness, and coughing and gasping. The drugs we prescribe are strong, but don't seem to be working at all.

Shona has been admitted again, more sick than ever. The doctors have suggested reducing her treatment regime of aggressive antiretroviral drugs in the hope that the side-effects lessen. But Empress wants to continue with the high dose, at least for a few weeks: 'one last try'. The ward's clinical nurse educator, a Liverpudlian woman named Emma, tells the doctors that compromise is in order: Shona should be allowed to continue on her current antiretrovirals as well as IV antibiotics for the next week. Emma knows the family inside out. She has cared for Shona for many years, and when the extended family visit, carrying pots of food that they are not supposed to eat in the hospital cubicle, they hug Emma as though she, too, is a relative. Emma ushers them and their contraband in and doesn't mention the smell of stew and Scotch bonnet as it wafts down the ward. All patients have favourite nurses. And all nurses have favourite patients.

Shona's side effects do not worsen, and she recovers a bit – thanks either to the antiretrovirals or the antibiotics – and Empress does too, thanks to being listened to and having some power over her daughter's care. Nurses calculate risk and see the big picture. Medicine can be rigid in our Westernised model of care, but nursing can be fluid, able to bend and shift; and, with it, nurses sometimes change their own thinking and understanding, too. While I am learning so much from my nurse colleagues, I am learning even more from patients and relatives. Empress is the kind of parent I'd like to be one day, at once both fierce and gentle. I always imagined that being a nurse was about caring for patients. It turns out that caring for the families of patients is the tricky part, the unseen creative nursing that often makes the most difference. Perhaps palliative-care nurses understand this the most.

When my dad is diagnosed with incurable cancer, I phone my friend, Aliyah, a palliative-care nurse who is a clinical nurse specialist in oncology in the north-east of England. I am at that stage of the process when I think I can fix everything: get the right treatment, a drug trial, a second opinion, a different opinion – the right one. I am not ready to accept that my dad will die, so I channel my every waking moment into fighting. I talk to specialists, google everything and spend hours on the phone trying to get his oncology appointments moved forward. Every day counts. Every hour. I imagine the tumour inside my dad growing as time shrinks. I imagine him unable to breathe, and afraid. I will not let myself cry. I need to fix this. I *can* fix this.

I ask Aliyah many, many questions and she listens carefully to them all. She has in the past described her job as the most creatively rewarding of all areas of nursing, and now she gives me ideas of ways to prepare for his death and for his absence: memory boxes, video clips to show the grandchildren, asking my dad to write letters, writing him letters. I am not ready for any of this. I focus instead on the science: the exact combination of drugs that my dad has been prescribed, and the alternatives. Aliyah listens as intently and warmly as ever. She offers, in a heartbeat, to travel and see me, despite having four children and a full-time job. 'There's nothing you can do,' I tell her. 'There are always things people can do,' she responds.

Like all the palliative-care or bereavement nurses or family-support nurses I've worked with over the years, Aliyah is full of goodness to the core. She reminds me that all of us are so much more than blood and flesh and bones. She sometimes speaks in riddles: 'We are divine, each and every one of us, with stories that go on.' At other times she is straight-talking. After listening to me speak about my dad – phone call after concerned phone call – and after asking how I am coping, she pauses, then asks how my mum is. She almost has to shake me into truly understanding the situation. 'It's the person who is left behind who suffers the most. Always.' She isn't talking about me, I finally realise, after selfishly thinking she is. And I hear what she is trying to say: my dad is sick, and coping with that – the struggle of every hour, the pain and the admin of having cancer – is all-consuming. He's distracted by simply trying to be alive. At last I see it: my mum is suffering a far-worse pain. And her pain will not end with my dad's death; there will be no rest or peace for her. Aliyah helps me to understand that it is the living who hurt more than the dying. It is my mum that I need to hold up.

Initially my mum is in total denial, as am I. When neither of my parents speaks about the practical plans of dying and funerals and cremations, I wonder if my dad's cheerfulness is a way to protect my mum from his pain. If it is, then it seems to be working. She delights in it. My dying dad is better at holding my mum up than I am. He doesn't talk of pain or sadness, but instead focuses on his two favourite things: food and gambling. My dad's primary concern, after family, is to continue to enjoy his dinners, and to keep going to the casino for as long as possible. This may make him sound rich, but he is not. My dad bypasses the betting tables every time and sits at 'his' fruit machine, which is in the shape of a toucan, the tropical bird. Although in no way a spiritual man, he is incredibly superstitious, which must be a shadow from his mother, who is a spiritualist and regularly has conversations with dead people. *This* is the only machine in the world. He sits with a pint of beer, or a large whisky, and puts coin after coin into that machine. Occasionally it makes a shrill bird sound, then empties some of my dad's coins back to him. His face could not be more delighted in those moments. It is beautiful to watch, for he is so completely and utterly in the moment, not spending a second thinking about cancer or death.

My dad is so good at dying, yet now that the clock is running out he wants to live more than ever. One day he comes home from the casino much later than usual, and very sad. I'm staying with them. My brother and I regularly get a phone call or text to say he's taken a turn for the worse and we need to get there quickly. We fly over to the Isle of Man, tearful and panicky, only to find him sitting up in his armchair eating, of all things, roast goose, or Staffordshire oatcakes, or going through the racing results in the newspaper, getting excited about who he will put down for £2.50 on the nose: 'Whippersnapper has it today! Happy Girl is looking lively, too.' And my mum potters around, busying herself caring for him. She wants to nurse him at home, they have decided. It's difficult to think of my mum as a nurse. Caring for dying people at home is hardly ever what is imagined. I am worried for them both.

Today, though, my dad's not bouncy or excited or grinning about food or gambling. We have been warned by his nurses that he'll be up and down and that this is okay, but it's heart-breaking to see him feeling low. I take a deep breath in the kitchen and then walk into the living room with a cup of tea for him. He looks at me with sad eyes and I try not to focus on the greying of his skin, the skinniness of his body. I smile and sit next to him; put his tea down and lean against him. His smell is the same as ever: oranges, cigarettes, wood-smoke.

'Can't believe it,' he says.

'Maybe the shock is sinking in,' I say. It's been weeks since he was given the bad news. He's still taking palliative chemo-therapy, but more to stop the awful symptoms than anything else.

But he looks at me funnily. He then explains that when he went to 'the cazzy' there was a woman playing *his* machine. 'Bloody toucan,' he says. 'And she won.'

He plays that machine right up until his death and never wins more than a few pounds. But he also bets on every single thing you can imagine. He and his friends sit all day in the pub, betting on horses or dogs, or whether or not the next person who walks in will be fat, or whether a wet matchstick will stick to the ceiling. Every single thing. Dying means different things to different people. For my dad, dying means living it up – in his own way – until the last possible second. It is not a time of sadness for him, but a final roll of the dice: winning or losing, and a slap-up dinner either way. I believe he does that – lives that way, and dies that way – for my mum. We don't discuss anything philosophically. But we watch a football match a week before my dad dies, and his team scores in extra time.

He grins at me. 'Amazing what you can do in those final minutes,' he says. 'Extra time.'

Like my patients, my dad teaches me that hope can exist, even in the darkest of places, because we are human and destructive and beautiful. And we have love. I remember the words of Empress. *Faith is not knowing. It's hoping.* Death is never the end. Nobody ever really dies. Not if they are loved.

Shona turns seven by the end of my placement, after I have failed and resat my final exams. I can still see her. Despite being small for her age and developmentally delayed, with partial paralysis and hepatitis, she is completely unafraid as she sits on Empress's lap with an oxygen mask. I notice her breathing is shallow, but I know there is a doctor on the way to assess her. I am administering her a blood transfusion and have a large white plastic tray, on which sit the pouch of red cells, a saline flush, a blood giving set, an alcohol wipe and a pair of sterile gloves.

I have begun cleaning her IV line when Shona speaks to her mum, her voice muffled behind the mask. 'I can see them, Mummy. Those lights.'

I stop what I am doing and lower the oxygen mask a fraction. 'What lights?' I'm worried she might be suffering from neurological symptoms that indicate a medical emergency. I'm on high alert for subtle signs. But Shona seems fine. Her pupils are equal and she's recognising me.

'The lights,' she keeps repeating. She smiles. 'All around my head.'

Empress strokes Shona's neatly plaited hair and sings. She rocks her back and forth.

It is a week later when we know for certain that Shona will not survive. All the drugs have been stopped. Empress sleeps in the room next to her bed, a mass of hospital blankets and the smell of sour sweat covering them both. Shona spends her days cuddled up on Empress's lap, drawing picture after picture of flashes and glowing lights, leaning her head towards her mum's chest and breathing in deeply, as if the sour-sweat smell of her mum is the nicest smell in the world.

'I can see them, Mummy,' she keeps repeating. 'They are everywhere.'

Empress holds Shona in her arms and tells her she can go. It is time. She spends an entire day telling her. 'Go home now, Daughter,' she keeps repeating, over and over again. 'I will come and find you one day soon. Go home now.'

Later I walk past the side-room and I cannot hear any singing. No more Empress telling her daughter that she can go. I know what must have happened. Shona is DNACPR – not for resuscitation, should her heart stop. But the staff have asked Empress to call them if her breathing worsens, so they can be there to support her. But Empress is the sort of woman who would not call a nurse or a doctor when the time comes. Because she is the only person who matters in that room – the only one important to Shona. They belong to each other, not to us.

I open the door a fraction to see them both on the rocking chair, Empress looking down at Shona's quiet body. A thousand dancing fireflies pattern the wall, the ceiling, where Shona's drawings are displayed. The room is filled with light. Shona is gone, but she is everywhere.

'He asked for a satsuma just before he died.' My mum is lying on the bed. 'Even though he couldn't eat by then. He wanted to hold it.' I am lying on my dad's side, in his imprint where he died; it is strangely comforting and surreal. My mum has taken a small, shrivelled satsuma from her bedside table and is sniffing it. She holds it up to me. 'This – this is the satsuma.'

It is the size of a walnut and has grooves all over it, like an elephant's skin. It reminds me of my daughter's Mongolian-spot birthmark the day she was born, which always feels like yesterday, no matter how the years roll by. She is permanently a baby, in my mind, no matter how old she gets. I must be like that to my mum. 'You kept it?'

By now it is four years since my dad died. Same mattress. Same satsuma.

My mum sniffs it again. 'The exact one. I sniff it last thing at night and first thing in the morning.' We both look at each other for a few seconds, unblinking. 'Your dad would have said I've lost it.'

'Nope,' I say, pressing my body into the mattress where he slept. 'He would have said you're fucking crazy.'

Then we burst into laughter, and we laugh and laugh and laugh, a thing I would never have thought possible in the very bed where my dad died. All thanks to a satsuma, and my mum's understanding of what it represents: my dad's absolute love of life. Even during 'extra time'. He reminded me of what nursing has always taught me: that this life, this human condition, is full of wonder and awe. We are made up of golden light, sunsets, dawn, and the before and the after. How precious this thing is that we can't really put into words, or art, or music. There is so much we can't understand; and perhaps we're not meant to. Maybe this is acceptance?

Later that day we go to the casino, drink a whisky and visit the toucan. My mum studies the machine as if there's a formula to learn. We frown, trying to understand. She sips her whisky. I down mine. We both hate whisky. I put my hand on her shoulder as she puts a coin in, then pulls the lever. The toucan makes a squawking noise. And I hear the sound of faith.

We don't win. We never win. But we smile anyway.

2

Cows that Jump Over the Moon

I am on a short placement with a district nurse and cannot wait to get back to the hospital. My friend has her first placement in Accident and Emergency (A&E) and I'm jealous, hearing her stories of cracking chests and resuscitation. I am eighteen, arrogant, enormously naive and, at times, unkind. I follow the district nurse around, reductively imagining her job: dealing with wounds, leg ulcers, colostomy bags and incontinence. In her bag, instead of emergency equipment, are bandages and dressings. 'This particular dressing pulls out the pus,' she says, holding up a packet. I smile and pretend I am not horrified.

Sylwia (pronounced 'Sylvia') is from Poland and her accent has hard edges, despite the words being soft. She talks a lot: about her lovely patients, the height of the snow in Poland at Christmas, and her husband, who is working five jobs – carpenter, gardener, early-morning cleaner, handyman and oven-cleaner. 'In Poland,' she tells me, 'my husband had a successful business as a builder. He sometimes will come and fix my patients' sinks, toilets, handrails on his days off. He is a good man.'

I am sure it is against the rules to let a husband act as handyman for her patients, but I don't say anything.

The first house that Sylwia and I arrive at is the home of a sixty-four-year-old with Parkinson's disease, who has recently been discharged from hospital having suffered community-acquired pneumonia. He needs antibiotics and on-going treatment for the severe pressure sore he developed in hospital. As well as her usual bag of nursing kit, Sylwia is carrying a small red heart-shaped balloon. James is bed-bound and looks extremely unwell. But when he sees Sylwia and the balloon he shrieks with laughter. Sylwia ties the balloon to his bedframe and kisses the air above him. 'Happy Valentine's.'

James beams, but it's hard to feel his happiness. Beneath the smile, his face is twisted in suffering. I scan his bedroom. It is neat and tidy, almost clinical, and there's a hoist next to his bed, the first I've seen in a domestic setting rather than hospital. He doesn't look as if he needs hoisting anywhere – he's emaciated and his skin is hanging off, as though maybe he was once big and lost weight too quickly. He's wearing a football shirt over pyjama bottoms.

'Chelsea! And I thought we were friends.' Sylwia puts her bag down next to the bed, reaches across and touches James's arm. 'This is Christie, she's a student nurse working with me today.'

I smile. 'Hello. I hope that's okay.'

James sort of shakes his head, then nods, so it's difficult to know what he means, but then he says, 'Sure'. He looks at the balloon. 'Beautiful. What a nice thing.'

'How have you been? Have you experienced any pain?'

'Just crawling and weird sensations,' he says. 'Bit of itching. It's strange.'

My feet feel as though they want to walk backwards and edge out of the door and the house, run into the road and away from nursing entirely. I focus on the balloon.

'Let's have a look then.' Sylwia washes her hands, opens a dressing kit, and then we roll James to the side of the bed. On his sacrum, at the base of his spine, is his pressure sore. Pressure sores are preventable and are a risk when a patient is unable to move. They can be fairly minor, like blisters, and heal quickly, or they can cause serious problems – a grade-four pressure sore may be deep enough that you can see bone. They are horrific reminders of our mortality – the weight of a body turned against itself.

We must keep moving or be moved, or we begin to die.

James has developed a grade-three pressure sore that is not healing. Instead it has become sloughy and is necrotising – dying. If it gets worse it could lead to necrotising fasciitis (also known as the 'flesh-eating disease'), Sylwia tells me, so something has to be done about it. She slowly peels away the dressing, and it is then that I see them. The maggots. Like tiny grains of rice. James's wound is the size of an orange and is alive with maggots. And it is the nurses who put them there.

Maggot therapy is not new. Napoleon's general surgeon, Baron Dominique Larrey, reported from Syria at the turn of the nineteenth century that certain species of fly only consumed dead tissue and helped wounds to heal. But maggots have been used since antiquity. 'The blowfly larvae – or maggots, if you want – help debride the wound. We only use sterile medical-grade maggots,' Sylwia tells me, as if she's describing any other medicine. She will have seen my pallor, though. 'It's very rare. This is the only time I've used them in ten years in the community. Special treatment for a special man.'

James turns his head to the side, smiles.

'I'll go and make tea,' I manage. 'If that's okay?' I need to get away.

James lies still, seemingly unperturbed. 'Two sugars,' he says. 'There's a cup next to the sink.'

The kitchen is immaculate too, everything bleached and polished. Almost too pristine. I wonder who cleans James's house, or if he somehow manages himself. I try and think of that, rather than the itching. I will never eat rice again.

'You need grit,' Sylwia tells me, in the car heading to the next visit. 'District nurses know better than anyone else that life is hard. And if you faint or something in front of my patient, I will tell your lecturers that you need to repeat your entire placement.'

Our next patient has suffered a fall and is ninety-four years old; he looks as thin and frail as a baby bird. He has a walking frame and sticks but, Sylwia tells me, has been sleeping in his chair. 'You can tell from yesterday's paper on the doorstep, Kayode, that you haven't made it out of the chair today.'

The double incontinence might also have given it away, but Sylwia doesn't mention that. Instead she puts a pillow behind his head and takes a long time plumping it up and arranging it for him. Kayode has a pained and embarrassed expression on his face, but Sylwia distracts him with her words and her fussing. 'Go and make some tea,' she says to me, 'while I clean this wound. And while the kettle is boiling, I'll give Kayode a quick wash, too.'

On Sylwia's list of patients are people suffering from heart failure, auto-immune diseases, dementia and numerous co-morbidities. She cares for oncology patients at the end of their lives who need palliative care and patients requiring home ventilation. People with every complex illness or disease you could imagine. But today, it seems, she is seeing patients needing wound care. My stomach is in queasy knots, especially after the maggots. But I try to suppress my light-headedness, and focus on what life must be like for poor Kayode and patients like him. What life might be like for all of us, one day.

It is so cold in Kayode's flat that I can see my breath. He is clearly unable to afford heating. I empty the kettle of its foul water and chunks of limescale, fill it and put it on to boil.

The fridge is bare of anything except a single onion, an opened can of tomato soup, a bottle of what I at first think is brown sauce but then realise is actually ketchup that must be ten years old, and an ancient pork chop on a plate.

Sylwia has already told me that many of her patients live alone and either have no family or one that is far away and doesn't visit. 'This wouldn't happen in Poland,' she tells me. I think about Britain in comparison to other countries. One friend from Ghana lives with two generations of his family, and they all take it in turns to cook and care for the grand-mother. Another friend from Italy recently moved back home to care for a sibling with cancer. I wonder why some societies care for their loved ones when they are older or sick, and why others don't. Whether it has anything to do with secularism.

When I return, with two cups of black tea, Sylwia has somehow managed to wash and change Kayode and is combing his hair, very gently. Kayode's face has relaxed a bit. I put the tea on his table. 'There you go.'

Sylwia looks at it, picks a cup up and slurps. 'Lovely cuppa,' she says.

'Thank you, love,' Kayode says. 'Thank you. I don't want to be a bother.'

'You're no bother at all,' she tells him. She darts into the hall and returns with the heart-shaped balloon she had left beside the door. 'From a secret admirer,' she says. 'Happy

Valentine's, Kayode.' And she leans over and kisses him on the cheek. Kayode looks as if he has won the Lottery.

Kayode has what Sylwia describes as poorly managed diabetes, which has caused blindness in one of his eyes, vasculitis and leg ulcers. He also has heart disease, kidney problems and is at risk of a stroke. Like so many patients, he has numerous comorbidities – or underlying health conditions. We may be here specifically to manage his diabetes, organise any changes to his insulin regime, perform complex assessments and re-dress his leg wounds, but despite Sylwia's level of skill and experience, she also offers Kayode the same basic care that is provided by his carers. She tells me later that there is nothing basic about care.

I watch her in awe. She first checks Kayode's blood-sugar levels and blood pressure. Keeping him out of hospital is a complicated process and, alongside Sylwia, he has meals on wheels delivered, visits from a physiotherapist (whose exercises Kayode apparently totally ignores) and an occupational therapist, who has organised handrails, and, as Kayode's hearing is not great, a special flashing doorbell. He also has carers who are meant to come in every day, but his carer has been off sick and it's clear, from the state of him, that they haven't been able to find cover for at least a week. Sylwia is a lifeline.

She kneels at Kayode's feet and opens her bag of dressings, before unwinding the damp bandage from his leg. I kneel beside her and watch. It's a huge dressing, and removing it takes many minutes. As she gets closer to his actual skin, the smell of his wound seeps out. Venous leg ulcers can smell awful. In preparation, I have put a smudge of Vicks decongestant under my nose, and I'm convinced Sylwia has noticed because she looks briefly at me, frowning. Kayode's leg looks patchy and raw, like the splashes of a burn, and there's a shiny discharge. For a few seconds my idea seems to be working: all I can smell is my childhood, when my mum used to smother my brother and me in Vicks at the first sign of the slightest cough. But then it hits me: putrid, foul eggs or prawns, or cat-sick or rotten cabbage, sewage, ammonia, sulphate, methane – all at once. My eyes begin to water. Sylwia simply ignores it.

She cleans Kayode's wounds as gently as she combed his hair, chatting all the while to distract him. She uses Hibiscrub, a pale-pink solution, almost bubble-gum colour, and dabs soaked gauze pads onto his skin with forceps. After that she blows on Kayode's legs, as though on wet nail polish, until they are drier, then dresses the ulcers, before carefully winding another bandage over and around them. When she's finished, Sylwia checks the bandage is not too tight, then smiles. 'Perfect!'

I'm trying to learn her techniques, but all I can do is press my stomach into a tight ball and focus on breathing slowly through my mouth, to minimise the stench. The full horror of nursing is beginning to hit me. The flesh and blood and bones of us all; the fragility of our human condition, which nurses must bear as part of their job. Am I cut out for it? This daily reminder of just how vulnerable we are?

After standing and shaking our legs out, after having kneeled for so long, Sylwia sets Kayode's ironing board up and begins ironing a shirt. 'You don't need to do that, love,' he says.

'While I'm here. And I'll contact our social worker to see if we can get you a fuel allowance.'

I look out of the window, through the stained yellow net curtains. It is cold and grey outside, and snowing lightly. I check the time. We have been allocated twenty minutes and we are now late for the next patient. I have no idea whatsoever why Sylwia is ironing a shirt, so I stand and hover. It is when Kayode starts chatting to her that I realise she is still nursing. She's treating far more than just his leg ulcers or diabetes.

Loneliness is a public-health epidemic. It causes about as many early deaths as smoking or obesity, and can increase the risk of high blood pressure, coronary heart disease, stroke, depression and cognitive decline. The charity Age UK reports that more than one million older people say they go for over a month without speaking to a friend, neighbour or family member.

Eventually Sylwia hangs up Kayode's freshly ironed shirt on the back of a chair, leans over and kisses him on the cheek again. 'See you tomorrow,' she says.

I'm sure that – alongside ironing shirts, and her husband fixing things – kissing patients is totally against the rules. But I watch Kayode's smile reach his eyes.

We get in Sylwia's car and I open the window. 'I don't know how you do it,' I say.

Sylwia looks at me. She starts the ignition. 'You have a lot to learn,' she replies. 'We will all be old one day. If we are lucky. You need to show respect, and if someone offers you a cup of tea, make an effort to drink it. If you can't, then pretend. Stay as long as you can. There is no disease in the world worse than loneliness.'

'I'm sorry,' I say sheepishly. I focus on the air freshener swinging to and fro from the rear-view mirror, and on the three other heart-shaped balloons in the back of her car. More Valentine's Day gifts for her patients, maybe. 'I just don't think I could make it as a district nurse. My mum is a social worker, and some of the houses she has had to go in ...'

'There's no better nursing. And it is an honour to work with elderly patients. You never know, I might change your mind by the end of this placement. You might choose district nursing,' she says, 'if you have enough oil in your head.'

I don't think much more about district nursing for many years. I don't think about Kayode for many years. But today I see his face, his fear, and think of his fall. I am crying and running through the hospital corridors to get to my nan before it's too late. She has fallen like Kayode did, and has broken her hip. Flashes of childhood accompany each of my footsteps. The day I turned up on my nan's doorstep after yet another argument with my parents and she said I could stay for ever, if I needed to. Her stories of living in Hong Kong and having new dresses made from beautiful silk, for a dance every evening. How I'd steal her Lambert & Butler cigarettes and smoke them in the bath, and we'd both pretend there must be a cigarette ghost. The times I cried and cried on her lap, even as an adult, and she'd rub my back and tell me everything would be okay – and I always felt I could believe her. She made everyone feel that.

Some families are patriarchal, but mine certainly isn't; my maternal nan, her mum before her, my paternal nan and a gazillion great-great aunts were all fierce, strong and modern women. One of them, Gladys, was so old it was hard to comprehend, and so small and shrunken that she reminded me of Yoda in *Star Wars*, yet despite this she kept a baseball bat behind her door, ready to kneecap anyone who dared try and burgle her flat. These women of my family, on both sides, seem to live, and fight, for ever. Except, now, maybe not my nan. She is old and frail and vulnerable. She fell over in the garden on a cold February night and broke her hip and was not found for hours. And she will probably die today.

I get to the ward and blurt out her name, but they have taken her to theatre already. She will die on the operating table. She is elderly, with multiple medical conditions. She was out in freezing weather, lying on the ground all night, in pain, calling out to the darkness. The thought of her being alone and frightened fills me up and hurts my bones, as though we are physically connected. Perhaps this is the worst of all things to suffer – the suffering of loved ones.

I turn a corner and there she is, on a bed, being wheeled towards the theatre, impossibly white and small, her grey hair flattened to one side, her eyes terrified and lonely. Her face is concave – they have taken her teeth out. She will hate that. This is a woman who, even now, gets her hair blow-dried every week. My nan can't see well, so I lean in close, grab her hand and squeeze it. 'Nan. It's me, Nan. I'm here.' And her face changes colour right in front of me, and I see that she can suddenly cope with anything. She's taught me how to make her feel that everything will be okay, in the same way she did for me.

But everything is not okay. Not really. The aftermath of the injury is worse than the event itself. And my nan is not alone in that. I learn much about broken hips – a fractured neck of the femur, in her case – and the fate that awaits many of us, particularly women, due to osteoporosis post-meno-pause. Hip fracture is the most common serious injury among older people. 'The wards are full of fractured neck of femurs – depressingly full,' a nurse friend tells me. 'All women of the same age and all now likely to die. The mortality rates after

33

a broken hip are shocking.' She tells me that one in three adults, aged fifty and older, dies within twelve months of a broken hip. I have no idea why. The research suggests an increased risk of additional complications, such as infection, internal bleeding, stroke or heart failure. The evidence also highlights a loss of physical function, increased dependence and decreased social engagement and quality of life. From independence to dependence: a sudden and total shift in one's way of life. Nurses know that 'giving up' is not a cause of death. Yet they also know that it is. You can die of a broken heart, despite what doctors will tell you. And you can die of a broken spirit, too.

My nan doesn't die. Instead there are mistakes and infections, and there is waiting. There are cancelled operations and a sense of complete hopelessness. We feel utterly vulnerable, and at the mercy of a failed system. It's the little things, too. Trying to get through to the GP. Spending hours waiting for an appointment, only to discover the ambulance wasn't ever booked. A pharmacist running out of a specific medication, and having to visit three other chemists before finding it. What do people without family to help them do? How do they cope?

My nan has gone from being a proud, active woman who washes her net curtains every week, tells random strangers at the bus stop about her family, makes enough cakes to fill a bakery and applies lipstick every hour, to being a frail, fragile elderly woman at the bottom of the social pecking order. She is house-bound and in pain. After one operation she is left with one leg shorter than the other; then in another operation they put metalwork in her, rather than replace the hip. It is quicker and it is cheaper. Nobody says this is temporary and cost-related. But I know the truth.

And I think about my nan's life. An army wife who lived all over the world, she raised four children. One son died at four, and up until the accident she still visited his grave regularly. She buried another son far too young. She had the best marriage of anyone I know. My nan and granddad shouted and laughed, and it was messy and full of noise and love; they had a red setter named Prince, which constantly jumped up between them. My nan has a house that is filled with my granddad, even thirty years after he died: the cupboards still stocked with his ginger ale, the radio still set to the shipping forecast, which he listened to devotedly, despite never owning a boat. Stories of my granddad weave through our lives.

But the memory that endures the most is when we were once on a motorway, my brother and me in the back of the blocky bright-blue Lada that made popping sounds, despite the fifteen-point check my granddad would insist on making before any journey, while my nan rolled her eyes. The horsebox in front of us contained, instead of a horse, a cow. A cow that seemed particularly agitated. 'That cow is going to jump,' my nan commented.

And my granddad called her bloody stupid, adding, 'Cows don't bloody jump.' Right before the cow, quite literally, jumped onto the bonnet of our car.

We swerved and there was a dent in the bonnet, and no harm done other than an escaped cow. My nan didn't say a word about it for the rest of the journey. That night my granddad sat making up stories for me, my brother and our many, many cousins. He always did, whenever we stayed with them. He'd sit on the blanket box outside the bedroom where we'd all squeeze into a shared bed, talking and giggling and doing silly dares all night. But we were quiet for my granddad. He was the greatest storyteller. We'd squash up, looking wide-eyed at the Artexed ceiling, and as his deep, rich voice floated into our ears, we would imagine entire kingdoms and universes. When he sang us Welsh lullabies – as, again, he did every night that we stayed – my nan would join in. The nonsensical stories were the best, though. He'd get all the folk tales mixed up. Cinderella would climb the beanstalk. Rapunzel would get eaten by a wolf. Sleeping Beauty would be disturbed by a pea underneath her mattress. And that particular night we all held our breath, as the cow jumped over the moon. He repeated the story. 'The cow jumped over the moon,' he roared. We children, from toddlers to teens, lay perfectly still in the darkness, huddled together, and listened to my nan and granddad howl with laughter. Theirs was the kind of laughter you perhaps hear only once in your life.

She could teach all of us a thing or two about the meaning of family, my nan. About the nature of love. And yet she is now frail and disabled, and vulnerable. She is afraid. I think of our elderly: our older people who all have rich lives and thousands of stories, like my nan. Those elderly patients we walk past in hospitals, in the community – almost invisible, and too often seen as irrelevant. Those men and women who fought wars for us, who risked their lives so that we might have one.

It is Dorothy, the district nurse, who saves us. My nan treasures her independence and is not overjoyed at the prospect of having a stranger in her house. She tells Dorothy she has enough help from family. She doesn't need a fuss, or a nurse. She is fine.

Dorothy is not easily offended. 'I'm all yours, no rush.' She speaks slowly and quietly, a pleasant change from everyone else, who seems to shout at my nan as though she is either deaf or stupid, or both. Dorothy picks up photographs before she checks my nan's prescription and her care plan, and scans the room for clues about her general well-being and health. About her life. 'Who's this handsome boy then? God, they look alike.'

My nan beams, proud. 'That's my grandson and his sister. He's adopted.'

She is talking about my son and daughter. I sit on the couch, flicking through the *Daily Mirror*, which my nan devours from cover to cover every morning. Whenever I visit, she will read out loud anything NHS-related, as if I must know personally the people involved.

I watch Dorothy look at the photograph of my children. It's true that they look alike, and they are closer than any siblings I've ever known.

'What a gift,' Dorothy says.

She must be stretched for time, but she never shows it as my nan describes first my son – how wonderful he is, and how much his sister loves him – then each and every grandchild and great-grandchild in turn. Once you get my nan talking, it is impossible to leave, for she too is a storyteller. She and Dorothy talk about politics (how the austerity cuts are destroying the world), the NHS (Bevin would be turning in his grave) and gravy (my cousin has brought home a girl who doesn't like gravy, which has made my nan extremely suspicious of her character and worried for his future). They laugh and laugh. They become friends.

When it's time for Dorothy to leave my nan, I can already see the change in her. For weeks she has been quiet and has somehow seemed smaller. Today she even has a stain on her top, which would have horrified her former self. But suddenly she seems brighter, as if the lamp inside her is not yet extinguished. She asks for a clean jumper and when she shouts, 'The cerise one, from Marks and Spencer', it's a huge relief, a comfort to me.

Dorothy performs all the nursing tasks she has to, and more, but almost in the background of their relationship, like a hairdresser who makes you forget they are cutting your hair. She is based in the GP's surgery and has a caseload of patients referred to her by the hospital discharge planning team, the doctor, the practice nurses and the patients and families themselves. She treats patients suffering everything from Crohn's to chronic obstructive pulmonary disease, and she delivers IV antibiotics, wound care, nebulisers, oxygen, insulin, rapid response and assessments of serious illness. She administers chemotherapy to cancer patients at home. She provides complex and holistic assessments to prescribe, deliver and treat people and their families in their homes and in nursing homes, homeless centres, refugee clinics and residential care settings; and, crucially, she keeps many people like my nan out of hospital.

Dorothy has assessed my nan's needs for equipment provision, mobility and independent living aids, and has given her information and guidance about her eligibility and applying for grants and welfare benefits. She has assessed and treated her physical, mental and emotional health. She does it all with skill, respect and tact. She has made my nan's entire life more bearable, at a time when it seemed unbearable. The job of a district nurse is increasingly complex, but at its heart it remains unchanged: to enable people to live – and die – in their own homes wherever possible, and with dignity.

She focuses on making my nan feel like the only person she is caring for, even though she has a busy workload, taking time to understand what treatment my nan needs and how best to deliver it. When she leaves, Dorothy blows my nan a kiss. And I remember Sylwia, and smile. And my nan beams.

'We really hit it off, me and Dorothy,' she says later. 'She's such a brilliant nurse. Makes such a good cup of tea.'

What a difference Sylwia and Dorothy make to the most difficult of lives. There is perhaps no starker reminder of our humanity than the work district nurses do. District nurses can see into the future, and it is all too often totally bleak. But they light up the darkest of skies. District nurses sometimes even become something like family, for those who don't have them. I spend my career working mostly in critical care, which is as far distant a speciality from district nursing as it's possible to get, though both jobs require equally high levels of expertise and skill. And all nurses teach me that whatever nursing you do, the single most important thing is that it is critical to *care*.

Some lessons take decades to learn, and something Sylwia said to me all those years ago finally sinks in: 'We are not alone, and nurses must remind the patient of that. Listen to your patients; they are trying to tell you something. Respect them.'

By now I know the Nursing & Midwifery Council (NMC) Code of Professional Conduct inside out. Sylwia was simply translating it into practice: it is in the smallest of actions that we can make the most difference for patients and families. District nurses remind their patients – and all of us – that when people feel most alone, and vulnerable, and afraid, they are not alone at all. We are not alone. And our elderly deserve our utmost respect.

Maybe I finally have some oil in my head.

3

The Taste of Lychee Jelly

My partner and I are in the adoption training centre, sitting in a circle with a group of other prospective adopters, mostly couples like us, with a board marker and a piece of paper each on the floor in front of us. We've been asked to list the things that led us here. *Miscarriage*, I write. *Hyperemesis gravidarum. Advice from GP not to get pregnant again. Wanting my birth child to have a sibling as close to her as my brother is to me. Hoping to do some good?* I would like to list the babies I've cared for who were waiting for adoption over the years. The children in the care system. The adults who suffer physical, mental and emotional problems as care leavers. Those who fall through the cracks.

I look around at the other lists. Some are long, but others are suspiciously short. The social workers are only worried when the list is too short. I know this. My mum is a child-protection social worker and we often discuss the prospect of adopting a child.

Social workers don't care who you are, I learn, or how you've lived or what you've been through. But if you're not able to be honest about it, or you have unresolved issues, then they are concerned. Children in the care system need therapeutic parenting, not simply good-enough parenting. Because they all have special needs. Social workers are far more interested in a person saying they want to adopt because they suffered years of IVF and now, after a period of counselling and grief, know it's the only way they will get to be a parent than if someone says they want to adopt because they think it's a great thing to do.

My mum is not the only social worker to tell me these things. Our own social worker, Teniola, is running the training session. She is wearing cowboy boots and a miniskirt and is eating crisps. I like her a lot. She's straight-talking and no-nonsense. Despite her support, the adoption training is still brutal. We learn mostly about child abuse. I know a lot of it, both from child-protection training at work and from first-hand experience of caring for babies and children who have been thrown against walls or beaten, or who have had to care for younger siblings since they were only four years old themselves, and other unbelievable horrors. I haven't, though, ever thought of it in the context of a potential child of my own suffering it. My imagined child. I think my imagined child must be a girl, and she will look like my birth daughter – partly because that's what my birth daughter keeps telling me. I picture the two of them, Afro puffs and smiles as we laugh together in parks and at the seaside. It's a fantasy of course, but a good one.

My daughter is three. It's hard to know how she will cope with any sibling, particularly a sibling with additional needs. But I try not to think of that, although the social worker forces me to. 'People have misconceptions that children are put into care. But they are almost always *taken* into care. Most often as a very, very last resort, and often after abuse, whether emotional, physical, sexual or neglect. Often a combination of all of those.'

We begin the course as strangers and end up knowing more about each other than some siblings do. The training takes place early on in the adoption process – I suspect to weed out those who will walk away, when confronted with the reality of it. On day two, three people are missing from the training and I never see or hear from them again. A woman named Poppy takes up most of our time.

'We really want a daughter,' she keeps saying.

Teniola is poker-faced. Like a nurse. 'Well, gender is one of the things you do get to choose. But we like to know and understand the reasoning behind it.'

There's a list of things you can specify that you will, or will not, accept in an adoptive child, ranging from serious medical conditions to one occasion when a social worker asks us, in all seriousness, if we'd accept a child with red hair.

Poppy is dry-eyed as she tells this room full of people about the daughter she lost. 'She was born with her brain outside her head,' she says. There is silence, and the room is full of shadows. 'She lived for three days.' Her husband, Lee, puts his arm around her. Poppy shrugs it off. I notice, and I see Teniola noticing, too.

'We just want a daughter. Also, can you change the names?'

A man to my left and his partner both cough.

'I mean, some of the names of the children are pretty extreme. We don't want Chardonnay or Tiger, or something. Our daughter was Jessica, so we'd like to call her that.' She laughs. 'We've already got her name on a print in her bedroom.'

Her voice is hollow. I wonder if she's ever had therapy. I feel so much sadness for this woman, and the horror of loving a baby who is born in such a way, a baby who only lives for a matter of days. I wonder, most of all, what life would be like for that poor second Jessica. We find out later that the couple don't make it through the home assessment.

I look at the example of the form they will expect us to fill in. The tick-box of what we could imagine coping with as a family, my partner and I. His twelve-year-old daughter, who lives with her mum, but stays with us regularly. Our three-year-old daughter. Everyone in this room is signing up to the unknown, but only my paediatrician partner and I understand what that unknown looks like. Serious parental mental illness, schizophrenia, bipolar disorder, congenital abnormalities, heart conditions, oxygen dependency, sickle-cell anaemia, Down's syndrome, a history of violence, domestic violence, neglect, incest.

'Loss and grief always start the adoption process, however it ends.' Teniola looks at us. 'Our most important journeys travel backwards.'

I look at the box that says 'Learning disability'.

Jake is fifty-four, wears special boots that straighten his legs, often uses a wheelchair and loves painting sunflowers. He is bouncy and excitable. And he is in love. He wants to share a room with Grace, a woman in her forties who is almost entirely non-verbal. She uses something a bit like a Ouija board, pointing at letters with her eyes. In pre-technology days, this is a time-consuming and frustrating process for all involved, especially for Grace. A sentence can take thirty minutes. I sit with her while, around us, the staff have a meeting about whether it's appropriate to let Grace and Jake share a bed.

I have shaved my head and wear DMs. It is 1997 and I'm working in a residential home for people who have physical and learning disabilities. It is a sprawling place, a large mansion in Dorset, with residents' accommodation that nurses visit. We volunteers – I suppose around thirty of us – do the bulk of the back-breaking work. I am sixteen, have £21 pocket money a week and am blissfully happy, spending it on roll-up tobacco and large bottles of cheap cider. It is akin to a hippy commune; we all share rooms and clothes, and strep throat and probably chlamydia. We are young. I am militant about human rights and point out to anyone I can that these are adults and they can do whatever they want. My thinking is black and white, and far from subtle. But the managers ignore me anyway and call in Jake and Grace's elderly parents, as though they are children.

So much has changed in perceptions of disability since those days, though we still have so far to go. Then we viewed people with disabilities with fear, stigma and pity, and we worked with theories of 'social role valorisation' and 'normalisation' – essentially, attempting to align the lives and routines of people with disabilities as closely as possible to what was deemed 'regular'. It never really made sense to me to adapt the patterns of a person's life to fit society. Much better, I would wax lyrical to my friends, to adapt society so that it's completely inclusive and everyone can feel and live 'normally'.

It turns out that Grace is a more accomplished campaigner than me. She knows exactly what she wants and how to get it, and she knows how to play the system. She points with her eyes as I write down the words: *Jake – will you marry me?*

They are assessed by many, many professionals to make sure there is true consent. And then they are married a few months later, in the most joyful wedding I've ever attended, and the managers can only look on as Jake and Grace drink too much champagne and ask the carers to help them into the same bed for a very early night. They go on to carve out a healthy adult life, despite none of it being easy for them, and despite living in a centre where they depend so much on the care of others.

Breda is living with her sister Bernadette and has avoided a care home. But they are finding things difficult. Their parents used to help with Breda, but they are elderly now. Their mum has dementia and is being cared for full-time by their dad, but he has heart disease. Breda has autism, which is defined by the National Autistic Society as a lifelong developmental disability that affects how a person communicates with and relates to other people and experiences the world around them. It is a spectrum of challenges, and Breda's autism is at its most challenging end. She bites and spits and is known to self-harm. She also suffers from pica: eating non-edible things, in her case, cigarette butts and soil; and she smears – which means wiping faeces – on the walls and windows of their shared flat.

Bernadette, having cared for Breda over the last eighteen months, suffers from an eating disorder and depression, and is on sick leave from her job as an administrative assistant. She's single: she has devoted her life to caring for her sister and has neither the time nor the energy for a romantic relationship. As with all patients, there is a giant jigsaw around them, and Breda's autism is only one part of it. These are the people whom nurses care for, the puzzles for which no textbook can prepare you.

Breda, on top of everything else, has severe asthma. And I think of all I've read about asthma: how the examples of caring for people make assumptions that the person suffering asthma is compliant, without additional needs or complicated family health situations. Increasingly, however, it seems that our patients arrive, like Breda, in a tangled ball of needs: social, emotional, physical, mental and learning challenges. A nurse is the one who sees the big picture that sometimes makes the presenting condition – in this case, asthma – treatable. Nursing is not so much about untangling lines as it is about untangling lives.

I first meet Breda and Bernadette one day in March on the ambulatory care ward. March is traditionally the month when the hospital – and its patients – is coming to the end of the respiratory-illness season and can begin to breathe again. The winter crisis eases slightly and nurses can, for the first time since October, start to see light on the horizon. March also often signifies the end of pneumonia and bronchitis and exacerbations of underlying conditions. And there are fewer elderly broken bones – no icy ground to slip on. Instead it is chickenpox season, when those children and adults with bad enough cases of chickenpox or shingles end up in hospital and have been among the sickest patients I've ever cared for. And it's the time for childhood accidents (I always wonder if children, having been cooped up all winter, suddenly go wild on their bikes or climbing trees). March, along with every month, is also for sepsis, cancer, dementia, heart attacks and those unexpected events that can leave someone permanently damaged. Asthma attacks can happen at any time, but in winter they are more common; and asthma goes hand-in-hand with other respiratory illnesses such as pneumonia, the two linking up and then bringing out the worst in each other, like badly behaved best friends.

Breda has asthma attacks throughout the year, many of them causing hospitalisation. She is having one now and needs a nebuliser, but she is also biting and spitting at the nurses and, as she's obese, is pushing away Bernadette with relative ease. I notice the expression on Bernadette's face. It's beyond tired or combative. It's as if she's just been told she is dying, and there's nothing more anyone can do. All hope is gone. A nurse standing with the nebuliser is wearing an eye visor, presumably in case she gets bodily fluids in her eyes. I think back to the eye washouts I've had over the years – litres of saline poured onto my eyeballs to flush out whatever blood or phlegm or faeces has ended up spraying towards them.

I see at once that Breda is struggling to breathe. The nurses have moved away as much equipment as they can, pulled the curtains and placed pillows around her bed, but none of it is helping. In between spitting deep-down guttural phlegm at the nurses and her sister, Breda is banging her head and eyes, smacking her face in distress. She drags her nails down her cheeks, drawing blood. Her oxygen saturation probe was flung off long ago, and her monitoring and cannula were pulled out. She is breathing inadequately, struggling with deep respirations, resting between violent bouts with her arms stretched straight in front of her. This tripod position seems to happen almost subconsciously to people in respiratory distress, when the body attempts to maximise lung capacity, using the accessory muscles of the neck and upper chest to draw more air into the lungs.

Our lungs are proportionately larger at the back of our bodies than at the front; this is one of the reasons why neonatal nurses lay babies prone. This applies equally to adult patients, though I have not seen this best practice widespread in adult intensive care – until now. Suddenly Intensive Care Units (ICUs) everywhere are full of prone adults, all struggling with COVID-19, all lying on their fronts, all receiving high PEEP (positive end-expiratory pressure) via ventilators and similar treatments. These adult patients remind me of giant neonates – all wrapped up on their tummies, pillows supporting them, in medically induced comas as we wait and hope their bodies will recover.

Tripod position is one of the red flags that tells a clinician the person is struggling and at risk of respiratory failure. For someone suffering with asthma, this is particularly ominous, as people with asthma can deteriorate incredibly rapidly. Breda is critically unwell, and beyond the nebuliser stage. I make sure the anaesthetist is on the way – and running. Breda will need early intubation with a breathing tube – endotracheal tube – and ventilation, or she is at risk of dying. Asthma is a devious disease. Life-threatening asthma has some subtle signs, and not being able to talk in a sentence is one of them, but this is impossible to assess with Breda's communication difficulties. However, her lips are tinged blue, which is a sign of imminent fatality in asthma. There is no time to lose. But any procedures will be near-impossible unless we can get a line into her. I step away from the bed, for the last thing Breda needs is another stranger amplifying her anxiety.

It's hard to watch. It must be so frightening for her, unable to breathe, in a strange place, surrounded by people wearing visors and PPE to protect themselves from her spitting, who do not know how best to communicate with her. Even now, as an experienced nurse, asthma scares me more than most other diseases. When people say 'asthma', most people picture an asthma pump or inhaler. Not so with nurses. I have flashbacks to patients I've looked after over the years with asthma: from fat, happy, wheezing babies laughing behind a cloud of nebuliser, to a teenager who died despite our very best efforts. Some air had become trapped in the wrong spaces on his body – a terrible thing called subcutaneous emphysema – and after he died I pressed my hand on his chest and tried to deflate him manually, so that he would not look different for his parents. His skin made a fizzing, crackling sound, like popping candy. When his parents came in, I remember wishing so hard that

I'd got rid of all the air, so that they might be spared the horror of that noise and sensation. However, his mum screamed and wailed so loudly there was no chance of anything else being heard. And I realised those sounds would have done nothing to their pain anyway. They had lost their son; nothing in the world could have made them feel worse. 'Asthma,' his dad said to me. 'It was only asthma and a viral chest infection.'

I run now to A&E, where I know there is an EZ-IO drill. Developed in the military for soldiers who have had their limbs blown off, this is a tool that drills into bone and can put an intraosseous line into anybody in a matter of seconds. It can even be used on conscious patients, although I would not volunteer for it. Despite the claims that it doesn't hurt going in, the very first flush of saline will be excruciating. There's a kind of mesh behind our bones and, while the drill doesn't disturb it, fluid splits it open, and that splitting will certainly be felt. But if Breda crashes, we will need the drill. Everything in A&E is behind glass and requires a code, like a vending machine, and it takes me a few minutes to find a member of the regular A&E staff who can access it for me. I run back to the ward as fast as I can.

My heart is in my throat by the time I get back. I want to help, yet I feel useless. I keep thinking of the boy we couldn't save: the feel of his distorted skin, the sounds of crackling and popping. But along with the drill, there is another unexpected lifesaving piece of equipment: Breda's care plan.

Breda has a specialist learning disability nurse, called a 'community behaviour specialist', and Bernadette has given the nurses a *positive behaviour support plan*, which details how she copes and the things that might help during episodes of challenging behaviour. When I get back with the drill, the bedside nurse has contacted the learning disability safeguarding nurse to make him aware of Breda's admission and has read through the care plan, which she hands to me. I scan the document while we wait for the anaesthetist, and it turns out that what Breda hates – and finds really distressing – are bright lights. Darkness makes her feel safer. I tell the nurses and as soon as we dim the lights, Breda stops spitting. She leans forward, resting on her outstretched arms, and her breathing becomes more effective. It's a small change, but it keeps her alive until the breathing expert arrives, an anaesthetist I know who modestly calls herself the 'gas woman'; and yet in truth she is one of the safest and most experienced pair of hands around. I feel my heartbeat slow as Breda is wheeled to theatre for a planned gas induction, intubation and treatment for her life-threatening asthma. Against the odds, she survives. I wait with Bernadette outside the anaesthetic room, and she leans on my shoulder. She doesn't cry. She's beyond crying.

'You're so brave,' I say, and Bernadette turns to me as if I have said something silly.

'I'm not brave at all. It's my sister who is the brave one. She inspires me to carry on, every day.' She looks at the door to the anaesthetic room. 'I wouldn't be without her.'

Even the most difficult lives are often full of love and laughter. Lucas has the most severe disabilities and yet he spreads happiness to all his family. Lucas dreams in music. He is ten years old, though he looks a lot younger as his body is much smaller than it should be. He has a twisted and turned spine, and his limbs are stiff and misshapen and contracted. He needs regular anti-spasm medication, and massages help, too. At the moment his wheelchair is broken and while he's waiting for a funding document to get the new one, he's in a spare chair. It's not a great fit, meaning that he's at particular risk of marks, blisters, redness and pressure sores. Lucas likes bubbles and singing and Disney films and rock music. If he screams, sometimes it helps to stroke his forehead. His swallowing difficulties mean that he can't take any liquids, and the speech and language therapist has advised that he also avoid solids at the moment. He is fed directly into his stomach via a gastrostomy button. Loud noises make him jump. He loves horse riding and, once a year, goes on a holiday organised by a children's charity.

This is the information I have about Lucas before I meet him. I am working in the community as an assistant manager of a residential respite centre for children with profound learning disabilities. Documentation is such an important aspect of nursing, yet it is much groaned about. But it's essential for children with needs as complex as Lucas, moving as he does between services, in and out of hospitals, and with so many different people involved in his care. His learning disability nurse, Tina, coordinates his care, linking into a whole the bits of information passed between everyone involved: school nurse, social worker, community paediatric nurse, speech and language therapist, occupational therapist, physiotherapist, teacher, teaching assistant and dietitian. If it takes a village to raise a child, then it takes a city to raise a child with special needs.

Tina is at the centre of it all, a magician, performing tricks that can't be seen in order that Lucas and his family can experience pleasure – or, at least, less pain. Tina has been diagnosed herself with an autistic spectrum disorder. 'For a long time, I thought about being a nurse researcher, and I was going to do adult branch,' she tells me. 'But when I found out more about learning disability nursing I knew I'd love it.' Like all nursing, learning disability – or intellectual disability – nursing requires creativity, adaptability and a huge dose of common sense. 'I go to work every day with one aim: to make people's lives better,' she tells me. She has been a learning disability nurse for many years in many settings. 'Sometimes that means sorting out new medication, or respite care, or accompanying a client to the dentist, so I can explain things in a way they understand. And sometimes it means attending a speed-dating night, to make sure everyone is having fun and staying safe. Or teaching a group of GPs about best practice. It's so varied. It's the best job in the world.'

Tina is the kind of nurse we'd all want: experienced, unafraid, determined. She fights for the rights of the people she cares for, within a system that too often doesn't seem to care for them at all. She teaches me so much – and I need the help. I'm green around the gills, early twenties now, only a few years' nursing experience, with almost no real-life experience. Many people go into learning disability nursing later on in life. It's not glamorous. There is no place for adrenaline-junkies. When I start out in nursing it's the high-tech, fast-paced, life-and-death world of hospitals that excites me. Yet while this nursing is quieter, it is by no means smaller. As a nurse, I am learning how powerful it is to save a life. And I am learning how powerful it is to give meaning to a life. Both actions save lives, in the end. But the latter saves many lives all at once.

'Every single human being deserves to live with dignity and be allowed to express happiness, sadness and choice,' Tina tells me. Positive relationships and delight can be found, with the appropriate care, expertise and financial support, to help not only those with PMLD (profound and multiple learning disabilities) or autism and challenging behaviour, but their families as well. The simplest things can have a serious impact on improving quality of life: the right assisted-technology communication aids, person-centred planning and a package of care and support. The right nurses. Learning disability nurses such as Tina understand the capacity for joy in all human beings. They know it gives meaning to the most difficult lives. Noam Chomsky said, 'When we study human language, we are approaching what some might call the "human essence".' Learning disability nursing is the study of a language that has been diminished and vilified, and disregarded as lesser. These are the nurses working in the field of human essence.

Tina described Lucas to me as a lovely soul, and I see it at once. Lucas shudders almost continuously, as if in pain, but also smiles with his eyes. It makes my eyes smile too, just looking at him. He is non-verbal, but does make noises and snorts and sometimes screams. His parents are unsure about his ability to process sights and sounds. 'I think he knows we are there,' his mum says. A cloud passes across her face. 'I think. Well, I hope so.' She picks up her son's hand and kisses it. Then looks at it. 'Let's cut your fingernails, Lucas.' She turns to me. 'He can scratch himself. Or other people. We try and keep his nails super-short.' I notice scratch marks on her arms, and old silver scars. They remind me of the silverfish that completely covered the carpet of a dark, damp flat I once shared with another nurse, after moving out of the nurses' home, where we had a stage-prop coffin instead of a coffee table, which we found discarded outside the London Dungeons. We thought it would make a good talking point, and we couldn't afford a coffee table.

'I can do it. If you want to go?' I offer.

The children at our residential respite centre come in with significant care needs, and the centre is designed to allow the parents of caregivers a much-needed break. These children do not have life-limiting diseases or illness, they will grow to adulthood, but they will be reliant on care from others for ever. The unit is a bungalow at the end of a long drive in suburbia. The neighbouring houses are privately owned and the people living there barely interact with us at all – staff or clients – except when the minibus is blocking the drive. Some of them have children, and yet they are kept away, separate from ours. They stare whenever we go out, openly and without any apparent shame, and sometimes I'll shout over, 'Come and say hi' or 'Come and play'. But my shouts are met with silence. Or fear. People can lack the courage to care.

The house has a large living area with hardly any furniture, so that there is room for wheelchairs; and there are no break-ables, so that any child who visits us can jump around, waving their arms as much as they want, without consequence. The bedrooms are off the living room, each bed with a ceiling hoist above it; they look like the claw-crane in machines at funfairs and motorway service stations, which are never strong enough to win a soft toy. Usually we don't bother with the hoists. It's easier for us to lift the children in and out of beds and chairs, and onto toilets and into baths. Of course I regret this now; we will all go on to develop back pain, and one nurse I work with ends up disabled herself, after many years of nursing, and is unable to walk or even sit without debilitating pain. There are many things I'd tell my younger nurse self, in retrospect, and to use the hoist would be high up on the list.

The kitchen is small and functional: tea and coffee for the staff, parents and caregivers, and a fridge containing the enteral feeds that most of the children have in place of food, via tubes directly into their stomachs. These large pouches of sour milk-like substance contain everything a person needs to stay hydrated and fed, including vitamins and nutrients. But they contain no happiness. There's food for those who can eat, and a variety of jellies for a girl who cannot swallow, but likes to taste. We make as many flavours as we can and she rests her tongue on them, then smiles. Her smile lights up the room and melts even the toughest of hearts. I am always on the lookout for unusual-flavoured jellies, and once in a Spanish supermarket I came across lychee jelly and almost screamed with delight, much to the bafflement of my travel mate.

I am learning about joy. For the children who can't eat, I try and use smell as a source of pleasure. I bring in different perfumes and candles and waft various smells in front of their noses, describing each in forensic detail, adding stories, as though this is a wine-tasting. This coconut vanilla candle reminds me of the first time I drank from a coconut with a straw, I tell them. The water is so good for you, hydrating, and it tastes slightly bitter, with hints of sweetness. Vanilla is the smell of Isle of Man ice-cream, where the queue in the summer for Davy's ice-cream stretches down the promenade in Peel, and in the background there's the castle, the smell of the sea and the sound of waves and happy children playing.

We use whatever we can to reach someone who is hard to reach. I bring in buckets of sand and put children's feet in them, so they can feel sand on their toes. We play tambourines and wave small musical bells beside ears. We make Rice Krispies cakes with the children – even those who can't eat – for the smell of chocolate and the sounds and texture. Caring for children with profound learning disabilities requires creative storytelling and sensory play. It means learning to think in new ways. It means learning a new language.

'Kunal's booked a restaurant,' Mia says. 'My favourite place. Italian. But really I'd just love to watch TV and eat a takeaway and sleep. Sleep – I haven't slept in so long. We don't sleep.' Lucas's mum, Mia, and his dad, Kunal, are leaving him here for the first time. But reluctantly. It is hard leaving any child, but leaving one with additional needs who can't easily communicate must be even harder. They live, like many people in cities, without any close family nearby, and have been reluctant to use respite care until now.

I can see the stress in Mia's face. But, mainly, the tiredness. Her eyes are eggcupped with grey crescent-moons.

'I understand. Why don't you tell him? He's probably as tired as you are.'

'It would break his heart. The first weekend we've ever had together since Lucas was born. He's such a romantic, you know. He proposed on Mother's Day when I was pregnant. Got down on one knee, but then sort of wobbled and fell.' She laughs.

Lucas doesn't laugh. But he hears her. His eyes widen a fraction and look somehow lighter.

She kisses his hand, then yawns. 'Sorry. I'm exhausted.'

I think about my friend who has a newborn baby and is sleep-deprived, totally exhausted, and says she can't wait to get to the six-month mark, when hopefully her son will sleep through the night. I think of another friend who is pregnant and obsessing about whether her child will inherit her 'strong nose' or her partner's 'musical ear'. 'We've put savings away already for a university fund. Or a gap year. Or a deposit for their first flat or car. It's amazing how much this bump is already costing me!' Expectations begin before we are born. I find it baffling that people imagine they will have a healthy and able-bodied baby and don't really consider any alternative. My worldview has been changed. Every day I see families whose entire life path has been diverted for ever, has gone on a totally different course. Opening your life to the possibility of a child is always wonderful. But it might not be at all what you think.

Mia tells me she watched every baby programme she could, read every parenting book, took every prenatal class. She drank juices and avoided all the right things – no alcohol or unpasteurised cheese – and ate organic vegetables only. But still she felt off-colour. And then one morning, after a holiday the week before, she woke up with contractions. 'He was early. Only a month, but still, I panicked so much because we just weren't ready. No cot. No nappies. Nothing. Honestly, I was so panicky.' She holds Lucas's hand again. I notice it is screwed up tight and twisted in hers, and Mia spends all the time she is talking trying to uncurl it a bit, to loosen the fingers digging into his palms. 'When he was born, Lucas didn't cry for a long time. I held my breath until I eventually had to breathe, then held my breath again. I did that four times before he cried. I remember feeling so relieved. Then I looked at the midwife's face. There was pity. She could see that he wasn't right.' Could there be anything more terrifying than a look of concern from a midwife? Scans can reveal many things, but not all. The technology is improving continually, but there are always things missed, because something changed, or it wasn't picked up, or it simply wasn't detectable on a scan.

Lucas sits with us as Mia talks. I ask her if we should perhaps talk in the other room, away from Lucas. And she laughs. 'He is here, but not really,' she says. 'He likes to hear my voice, but I don't think he has any comprehension of what I'm saying.'

We can't know that for sure, I tell her. Not really.

'I always wanted to work with nature. I was obsessed with flowers. We used to have lots of plans,' she says. 'So many. We had holidays and work, and cinema nights. We wanted three children, maybe even four. We're both from big families.' She wipes Lucas's mouth with a tissue. He has patches of soreness around his lips, angry red areas, most likely from permanent dribbling and licking his lips. Then she strokes his face. 'He is our whole life.' Mia's life is so difficult. She is up with Lucas every few hours. Every few hours for ten years. She had to give up her job as a florist and now can't work at all; she spends her entire life caring for her son, night and day, with some help from her husband, but little outside that.

'You need a break, though,' I say. 'He'll be fine here. We'll have fun, Lucas. I'll show you around and introduce you to some of the other children staying here, and the staff, and we can get to know each other.' I lightly touch his arm. He turns his head a fraction my way.

Mia looks puzzled that I'm talking to Lucas directly – something, I assume, that doesn't happen often. I am grateful for my training in children's nursing, with so much emphasis on communication; for children and adolescents of all ages, and in all situations. These non-technical skills, considered 'soft', are probably the most advanced skills of all.

'He likes you,' Mia says. She looks relieved. But she doesn't go anywhere.

'If you want to stay, that's fine, too. Whatever is most helpful to you. As long as you get a bit of a break.'

I leave the sitting area and walk to the bathroom, with another ceiling hoist above the bath and handrails everywhere, and the specially adapted toilet seat for the children who are not incontinent, although most of the children we care for wear pads their entire lives. I open the mirrored door, the shelves of which are lined with baby shampoo so that it doesn't sting eyes; talc to prevent rashes of all kinds; electric toothbrushes and different kinds of toothpaste. We try and buy a variety of toothpastes, from mint to bubble-gum flavour. Again these small, yet great, pleasures. I take out what I need and return to Mia and Lucas.

'I've got Vaseline,' I say. 'Do you mind if I put some on Lucas's lips? They look a bit chapped.'

Mia smiles. 'Oh, thank you. We usually have a ton of lip balm, but it's the one thing we forgot.'

I open the Vaseline pot. 'Lucas, this will help your mouth feel less sore.' I reach for his hand and, slowly, uncurl his arm. I dip his fingertip into the pot and bring it up to his face, help him dab the Vaseline around his lips. I close the pot and put it in the basket underneath Lucas's electric wheelchair, which is covered in stickers of smiling faces. 'You can keep this pot. We've got plenty.'

I turn to see Mia watching me. She looks at once surprised and relieved. She's sitting straighter and her face is less tired. 'I'm going to go, I think.' She stands up and gives Lucas a squeeze and a kiss. He flicks his head and rolls his eyes and snorts. Mia laughs. 'Oh, he always does that noise when he's happy. Don't you, Lucas?'

She kisses him a hundred times. Then takes a deep breath and leaves him with us nurses and carers. He watches the window for a long time.

'You have such a lovely mum,' I say. And Lucas snorts and turns his head. 'Let's make her a Mother's Day card.'

The following morning I have washed Lucas's face with a flannel and am now brushing his teeth. It's tricky. He keeps biting down on the brush and nearly onto my fingers a few times, but he doesn't seem at all distressed and I can tell, even in this short space of time, that his body language is as expressive as anyone's, despite the stiffness of his limbs. His head moves from side to side, and his fingers do not dig into his palms. I sing a silly song about brushing teeth and, as this seems to help him relax a little more, I continue. We finish in the bathroom and I am pushing him in his wheelchair to the hallway when the doorbell sounds.

'Who could that be, Lucas? It's pretty early.'

I open the door, with Lucas next to me, and find Mia standing there, in the rain, arms open. She rushes in and almost knocks me over. 'Oh, I'm sorry,' she says. 'I couldn't wait until three. I couldn't sleep.' She kisses Lucas's head and arms and hands, and his head again. 'My boy. My lovely boy.'

I let them have a moment, and smile. Nursing gave me the communication skills I needed to enable Mia to trust me with her son, to take the break they both needed so badly. It's impossible to measure the impact of that for her and her family, but I know it's profound. Before I disappear to put the kettle on, I look closely at her face: pure, utter joy. I look also at Lucas's face: pure, utter joy.

Their lives are difficult. Nobody signs up for this, or can even picture it. They live with daily struggles that most of us can't begin to imagine. And yet there it is in Lucas's eyes. On his mother's face. A reminder that love is love is love.

The adoption training room is full of fear, not love. I wonder how many people will make it through the training. I am not expecting to drop out, though. I have seen close up the most extreme suffering and the most extreme love. I know I have the capacity to love a child who was not biologically born to me: I love my partner's daughter. I care so much about her that I'd walk over hot coals for her, just as I would for my biological daughter.

Nursing has given me the gift of understanding the worst-case scenario in all things. But I also understand the bravery and unconditional love that families have for their relatives – that mothers like Mia have for their children. I look at the social worker going round the room with the example forms of the kind of children who need adopting. I scan the list of tick-boxes in front of me. And I know that when the time comes, if we get through the assessment, I will tick them all.

4

Making Pickles

In 2018 a former Russian military officer and double agent, Sergei Skripal, was poisoned with a Novichok nerve agent in Salisbury, alongside his daughter, Yulia. According to the *Guardian*, Abigail McCourt, aged sixteen, was heading home from celebrating her brother's birthday when she came across a man she thought was having a heart attack. She alerted her mum, Alison, and immediately administered first aid, undoubtedly saving his life. That Abigail's mother, Alison, is an army colonel and chief nurse did not come as a huge surprise to me. Military or defence nurses – and, by proxy, their children – are some of the most professional, compassionate and accomplished nurses I have worked with.

Military nursing is often thought of as something that happens in far-away war zones, and yet there is, and always has been, a network of defence nurses working in the UK in a wide variety of roles. There are around 5,000 medical reservists working in the NHS across the UK, and there is also a 'Step into Health' programme that recruits and trains former military personnel to become NHS workers. All nursing requires the ability to be calm under pressure, but military nurses are the experts at it. A bad day at the office is never as bad as some days they have seen, I'd imagine, and the steel that runs through them – the professionalism and confidence that their experience has built – makes for very safe hands in practically any circumstance.

After the publication of my previous book, *The Language of Kindness*, Fionnuala Bradley gets in touch to thank me for being an 'exemplary role model for the nursing profession', and I feel like a fraud. I'm always uncomfortable being seen as any kind of role model, and perhaps particularly so when, instead of doing the important work of these incredible nurses, I am writing from home, still in my pyjamas despite it being 3 p.m., and I have, in the last half-hour, managed to set the sleeve of my dressing gown on fire, frying halloumi. I am yet to even contemplate a return to clinical nursing. I suspect that, as Matron-in-Chief of Princess Mary's Royal Air Force Nursing Service (PMRAFNS), as well as Honorary Nurse to Her Majesty the Queen, Fionnuala – like most nurses in most settings whom I have had the pleasure to meet – is a far better role model than I am. She leads the 450 nurses of the PMRAFNS, known as the 'Flying Nightingales', who 'take pride in going where others cannot', delivering expert care and saving lives. We hear lots about soldiers, and rightly so, but I am yet to hear much in the mainstream media about the nurses saving lives in the most difficult of circumstances. Yet this team has been in existence for more than a hundred years, specialising in airborne evacuation from the battlefield back to the UK, providing critical care in the sky.

I am standing in the breakfast queue with my colleague, Xuan, the smell of fried bread making me nauseous. Today there are hot-cross buns, too. It is Easter Sunday. Nurses and doctors and healthcare workers miss out on Easter and Christmas, and school sports days and children's birthdays, without complaint. This is the job. Still, we make the best of it. The kitchen staff have put some daffodils on top of the counter, and a note is balanced against them: *Jesus is Risen*. And someone has scribbled underneath in biro: *Unlike Your Bread Rolls*. Xuan grabs a couple of hot-cross buns. She piles her plate high with sausage rolls and brown sauce and bacon and fried eggs, and I watch her, laughing. She may be tiny, but she deserves her nickname as the 'human dustbin'. She is also, as she tells me herself, 'strong as an ox', barely breaking into a sweat when performing effective chest compressions, even when a patient is super-morbidly obese.

I wait for the toast. The canteen has one of those ridiculous machines that are like a toast conveyor belt, which either burn or don't cook the bread at all. At least the smell of burnt toast overtakes that of the fried bread. Then I remember looking after a woman whose hair had got tangled up in such a machine and pulled her down towards the grill, scorching her face and ripping her hair out, and I remember how human flesh and toast smell almost the same, when burning. I am trying to push the memory away when the crash bleep goes off.

'Crash call for the neonatal, adult and obstetric teams. I repeat: crash call for the neonatal, adult and obstetric teams. Accident and Emergency. Ground floor, Cavell Wing.'

There's only one explanation as to why you'd need three crash teams at once: a heavily pregnant woman is in trouble. The adult team is to resuscitate her; the obstetrics team is to get the baby out (within five minutes, if either of them is to have any chance of survival); and the neonatal team is to try and resuscitate the newborn. Like all the other resuscitation nurses, Xuan and I are on all the crash teams – adult, paediatric, neonatal, obstetric and trauma – but this crash call will also bring specialist doctors: an obstetrician, a neonatologist, an anaesthetist.

We leave the toast, nodding to the kitchen staff on the way out, and weave our way, semi-running through the busy canteen. Much like ambulances trying to get through traffic, despite the alarms going off in our scrubs pockets, some people simply block our way. We push through the door and head down the long hospital corridor, which is always busy with too many staff, visitors, patients in wheelchairs, in beds, those bleeding, on crutches. One man walks past clutching his eyes. He has large bubbles and lumps on his skin, which look a bit like leprosy, but could be any number of conditions. We run on.

We run faster as the bleep goes off again, a third time, past the medical ward, where a family huddles together outside the door, their faces wet with tears; through the phlebotomy department, where people wait for hours on plastic chairs after taking a ticket from a machine; and outside the hospital as a shortcut: past the sexual-health clinic, where there is always a queue.

We speed up, past the hospital bins where smokers in their pyjamas and dressing gowns hold drip-stands and lurk underneath the sign that says *This Hospital Is a Smoke-Free Zone*; and past the meditation garden, where recently a woman tried to take her own life by drinking a bottle of bleach and there's a patch of dead grass where the bleach was spilled; past the MRI truck; the temporary crates, like shipping containers, that mark the hospital's attempt to meet the ever-growing demand; and an elderly woman in a wheelchair waving a cane to move a dead pigeon. We go back in through the staff entrance, where the swipe-access regularly breaks, and we are past the rheumatology clinics, where patients are having infusions of immunoglobulins and sometimes go into anaphylactic shock; past the cardiac outpatients clinic, where the cardiac technicians work – all of whom, in my own experience, look exactly like the genius technicians in Apple stores. They are incredibly intelligent, and sometimes socially awkward. I wave at Greg, the cardiac technician who has just been to resuscitation training and spent an hour trying to explain cardiac physics to a frightened-looking junior doctor.

We walk quickly past the long-term respiratory ward, home to patients who need ventilation for months and even years, their bodies sometimes deteriorating until they can no longer move at all. A patient describes his own muscular dystrophy to me as like turning very slowly into stone. A colleague once tells me, in all seriousness, 'If I ever end up on that ward in that state, unplug me.' A sign outside the ward has the National Health Service logo on it. Someone has crossed out 'Health' and written 'Illness'. Another has crossed out 'Illness' and written 'Suffering'. We stop a second: *National Suffering Service*. 'Pretty accurate,' I say, but I see a child's painting taped to the wall next to it: a tree made from colourful handprints, and the words *Thank you, NHS*.

I grab Xuan's arm and we're off again, faster now. We head down the back stairs and take a shortcut through the almost-always-empty basement, with the smell of chlorine from the hydrotherapy pool strong in the air. The palliative radiotherapy room has a few chairs of frail cancer patients waiting for this final treatment; and then on past the psychiatry offices and the finance department, the hospital kitchens and paediatric dentistry, and the endocrinology outpatients' clinics; and a large, impressive lecture theatre where every week there is a

Grand Round, discussing interesting or difficult cases; and the stuffy crash-trolley equipment rooms, where I've spent so many hours checking equipment and checking again – and where once, during an unusually quiet day, having told my manager about an information governance meeting, I had a nap on a crash trolley instead.

Finally we arrive in the A&E resuscitation area, and people are running in all directions. There are aprons and gloves flying around and there is shouting, and it's so hot and it smells of metal; it's always busy, but this is absolute pandemonium. Three crash teams, plus the regular resuscitation staff and A&E staff, and my eyes travel to the centre of it all, to the bed at the end of the room. A woman is split open right there on the ward, and a tiny baby is being pulled out of her.

Caesarean sections are usually performed in obstetric theatres, but in emergencies they can be performed anywhere. C-sections are usually performed by obstetricians with specialist training. But not always. I once attended the operation of a woman who was in a hospital that specialised in the cancer that she had. But she was also pregnant, so I was there with equipment to care for the newborn, should the baby need to be delivered. It transpired that there was no obstetrician there, and while the general surgeon may have insisted that 'anyone with a scalpel can cut a baby out, if needs be', I was not convinced. Luckily the operation went well and there was no need to test the general surgeon's theory.

This woman here is Suzanne. She's wearing a necklace, the hip kind from the online store 'Not on the High Street', which reads: *Mama-To-Be*. A leopard-print headscarf is holding her ombré hair back from her face. The rest of her is blood and gore, and flesh and insides. Her blood is darker than fresh blood should be. Oxygenated, healthy blood should be a vivid red; it takes my breath away whenever I see it. But Suzanne is wearing red nail polish that makes her own blood look dull.

Xuan clutches my arm. There are so many people that it's hard to know where to start, but the person in charge is a nurse with a military background, whom we know and respect: Amanda. She is one of the best nurses Xuan has ever worked with, a reservist who has worked in field hospitals in Iraq and Afghanistan. She's led many arrests and is always calm, efficient and friendly. 'Just because it's an emergency doesn't mean you can't find out the names of the team, and be nice. In fact it's even more important in an emergency.'

Amanda glances over and Xuan nods, so that she knows we're here whenever she needs us. We start tidying up, moving things so there's better access, working on the periphery and jotting down a handover sheet at the same time.

'RTA.' A nurse hands over the patient. 'Fractured pelvis and femur. No sign of the bleeding stopping.' Two nurses on either side of Suzanne hold up pouches of blood that they are squeezing into her, but nowhere near as fast as the blood is squeezing out.

I do not see how Suzanne or her baby can survive. I focus on the drops of sweat on Amanda's face, her eyes wildly searching for control, a plan – a way of saving this woman and her baby. Or at least one of them. I try and imagine the things she has seen and experienced in her military role. I am thankful that she now works in the NHS. I can't think of anyone better to lead such a horrific emergency.

'We need to get the surgeons, please,' she shouts. 'She needs to be in theatre as soon as we have this baby out. Like yesterday!'

A doctor is on the phone, asking for flying-squad bloods. In each hospital there are different names for ordering emergency bloods or blood products. Some are code red, or crash blood, which is simply packed red cells, used a lot in obstetric theatres; then there's massive haemorrhage or flying-squad bloods, which is all the goodies – all the blood products you need when someone is either bleeding to death or suffering a serious clotting disorder like DIC (disseminated intravascular coagulation) in sepsis. This parcel contains fibrinogen, fresh frozen plasma, cryoprecipitate, packed cells: all the by-products that blood contains.

I watch the defibrillator. Amanda asks a member of the team to put the pads on Suzanne's chest in advance of a surely imminent cardiac arrest. She's tachycardic and her heart rate is getting higher and higher. The obstetrician pulls the baby from her, lifts it out, vigorously wipes off the goo and places it on the resuscitaire, for another doctor waiting there with a miniature bag-valve-mask and a stethoscope, straight to the baby's chest. The obstetrician leaves Suzanne split open: it's impossible to see where the blood is coming from. Large gauze squares do nothing to mop up anything. Someone has put an incontinence pad on the ground to collect the blood-soaked squares, in order to weigh them and work out exactly how much blood she's lost, but there's almost no point. Anyone can see it's a devastating amount.

There are too many people around Suzanne's trolley and in the bed space. But despite the lack of room, everyone moves at speed without bumping into one another. Nursing, I understand by now, is not only anatomy and chemistry and pharmacology and law, but also anthropology, politics and sociology. Watching the team around Suzanne – each person perfectly choreographed by Amanda, the nurse in charge – their hands and arms and legs and bodies working at speed and doing different things, yet in some sort of synchronicity, I realise something else. Nursing is also dance.

Suzanne's husband, Simon, is standing outside the room. He's been waiting the whole time, a student nurse tells me, having followed her in the ambulance. I am not doing much good; the team of experts has taken over now, and Xuan and I are simply hovering in case we're needed. So I go outside and stand next to him. He's tall and bearded and has a kind face. His bottom lip is bleeding a little, where he's bitten it. He keeps opening and closing his hand, as if he has joint pain or is trying to hold onto something. I tell him who I am and that I'll wait with him while they are helping Suzanne. But he doesn't hear me, not really; he chats as if he's talking about someone else, or as if he's standing at a bus stop – as if being real and in this moment is simply too hard to bear.

'She's ordered a Bugaboo pushchair and is spending her pregnancy ordering everything possible from the Boden catalogue,' he says. 'I never imagined we'd end up as this couple.' He laughs a too-thin laugh. 'We met in a squat. Used to take the piss out of our middle-class parents.' He makes a loud noise as he exhales, as if he has no control of his breath. 'Now we are them. Everyone becomes their parent, sooner or later, right?'

He is looking at the door. His face is creased with pain. He jerks and his body looks as if it might topple over with stress.

'After ten failed IVF attempts and two miscarriages, we finally felt as if this one would stick around.' He looks at me, unblinking. 'She'll lose the baby, won't she? We'll lose the baby. I mean, it's too early. She was on the phone to me from the car. I mean she was hands free but still, she'd have been distracted.' He sobs. Covers his mouth with his hand.

I don't say anything. I don't know yet what he's been told and by whom, but it's clear that I'm not the right person, and this is not the right time to give significant bad news. Later I will replay the conversation and have a response: 'It's not your fault. They're doing their best; she's with the experts right now. Suzanne is seriously unwell, but the team is working so hard to help her and your baby.' But I'm terrified that if I open my mouth, the truth will fall out. And the truth – the terrible truth – is that they will probably both die. Not all babies live. Not all mothers live. Some births leave irreparable physical or psychological damage. Some women, it seems, despite their lifelong efforts, are not meant to be biological mothers. I've seen how much blood there is. Too much. I know the statistics for maternal cardiac arrest, if Suzanne loses output.

We stand in silence for a while, before finally I overcome the urge to cry or say nothing at all. 'Is there anyone I can call for you?'

He shakes his head. Nods at the door. 'She's my everyone.'

I nod. 'I'll pop back in and see how things are going.'

As I go through the door again I have to swallow down sick. I don't know this man at all and I feel under-qualified to give him any bad news. Giving bad news is something that I'm used to, but although it's considered a 'soft' skill, I think it's the most advanced of all the skills. It requires knowledge and some kind of existing relationship in order to be most effective. I need to know more about Simon than how much he loves Suzanne; and more about her than her burgeoning love for the Boden catalogue. In order to tell him the worst of all things imaginable, I want to know about his family, his support network, his history, his fabric: who he is and how he came to be that. But there is no time.

I look at the scene in front of me. The staff are covered in blood, as is the floor – everything. Suzanne looks barely alive in the middle of it all, a mangled mess of a human being, turned inside out.

I focus on the baby in the incubator. The baby is grey and small, and stretched out rather than curled over, as is normal. But the neonatologist looks up at the team: he gives us the thumbs-up. This baby lives. I exhale.

I rush out to tell Simon.

'They are working on Suzanne, and she's still critical. Everyone is doing all they can.' I pause. False hope is never good and I don't want him to underestimate how sick Suzanne is. But I can see that he needs something to hold onto. 'Your baby is alive.'

He looks at me in a kind of trance. 'I'm a dad?' he asks.

'You're a dad.'

And I imagine he'll be the best sort of dad. He is clearly so full of love. He doesn't ask whether the baby is a boy or a girl, and nor do I. Quite honestly, when things go this wrong, nobody gives a shit about those things that we usually obsess about.

Because pregnancy is not always healthy and happy. The UK now comes well behind many other EU countries in infant-survival rates, with twenty-four nations achieving better results. Inequality is widespread. Black mothers, like Suzanne, have particularly bad outcomes. Queen Mary University, London, reviewed thirteen studies from the UK, US, Denmark and

Norway, which found that black women are twice as likely as white women to experience stillbirth in these countries. And in the UK black women are almost five times more likely to die during pregnancy and childbirth than white women. This is part of why midwifery has become increasingly political and why fighting social injustice and institutional racism is – or should be – the vital job of midwives, and all healthcare workers. My midwife friend teaches me that supporting a woman giving birth is only one small part of her job, and often the easiest part. I am in awe of the work she is doing. Alongside her clinical work, she sees her job as driving political change, fighting oppression, championing girls and women. Being a midwife, I realise, is not simply about catching babies. It's about catching women.

Suzanne is somehow stable. She is placed in the high-dependency ward and her baby is on special care. I bump into Simon in the corridor, rushing between the two. He is carrying a soft-toy hippo. He looks like the happiest man in the world.

'Suzanne slept with the hippo against her skin. The midwife said our daughter can smell her, and it's the closest Suzanne will get to skin-to-skin for now.'

'Daughter?' I am smiling. I'm so relieved that mother and baby are alive and well and recovering. That's really all that matters about childbirth, in the end.

He's crying. Happy tears. 'I'm a wreck,' he says. 'She's so beautiful. Like her mum.' He holds the hippo as if it's his baby. 'She has these tiny feet and, when she yawns, this little scrunched-up face. I've turned into one of those baby bores who gets excited every time she moves.' He laughs. Then he bursts into huge, fat tears, a mixture of pain, trauma and relief. He tells me about Suzanne: how she didn't wake up for a long time, and it was the scariest moment of his life.

'We're thinking of calling her Amanda, after the doctor who saved her mum's life.'

I smile. 'Amanda is a nurse.' I imagine her face when she finds out. There can be no greater thank-you than that.

All day I'm smiling. And at the end of my shift I swing by the high-dependency unit to see Suzanne. She is sitting up, asleep but conscious, with a nasogastric tube taped to her nose and a central line sprouting from her neck. She has a large dressing on her chest, the top of which I can see above the hospital gown she's wearing. Her monitors all show stable numbers. I spot clues that tell me how well she's recovering: the lack of inotrope infusions, the single chest drain, the lack of ventilatory support, even the position of her bed – across the room from the nurses' station and crash trolley. All these things tell me that she's stable and will probably recover. It is amazing to see. Some people can survive anything.

This baby has a big story already, a powerful prologue. Mother and daughter will get to be together; Suzanne and Simon and Amanda will get to be a family.

*

Not everybody is that lucky. Today is going to be hard, my partner and I have been warned, but I am not prepared for how desperate it is. Of course it doesn't seem desperate on the surface. It appears like a normal children's party. We are in a church hall decorated with bunting, and there are folding tables set up with cupcakes and giant jugs of squash, and paper plates with Peppa Pig on them. But this isn't a normal children's party. On the way in there are giant boards on which are pinned leaflets advertising children. Each A4 sheet has a photograph of a child or group of children or a baby, then a short paragraph about what they like to do and what kind of family they need. It reminds me of Battersea Dogs & Cats Home:

> Harriet needs a home with experienced carers. She is lively and needs strict boundaries. She does not like to be left alone, and her foster carers describe her as a bundle of mischievous joy. Because of early life experiences, Harriet is unable to live in a family with other children or animals. She is making good progress and will make a wonderful, loving addition to the right family.

I try not to look at the papers, and we walk into the main hall. It should be a place of fun. There's a ball pit in the middle, and children of all ages, dressed in party clothes with colourful hair clips and clean faces, are playing and squealing. Older men and women stand at the edges with too-wide smiles, watching them intently while trying to appear casual. Foster carers, I assume, or social workers.

It could be any small child's birthday party, but there are cracks when you take a closer look. One of the children is running in a circle, getting faster and faster, and a woman is kneeling next to him, trying to calm him down. He is making a shrill, high-pitched noise and is totally ignoring her. Another baby clings to his carer, and as she tries to pull him away to put him in the ball pit, he grabs onto her clothes so tightly that he almost pulls her cardigan off, and she has to hold him close again. An older boy and girl stand together at the side, gulping down cupcakes, not with enjoyment but with urgency and fear. A young girl with an oxygen cylinder sits on a chair, watching the prospective adopters walk past her and reach down to play with the babies in the ball pit.

'Hello and welcome,' a social worker greets us. She is holding the leaflet relating to our family, as we prospective adopters also have photos and a blurb to interpret:

A mixed-heritage, mixed-faith medical and nursing family with extensive parenting and childcare experience.

Our experience puts us to the front of every queue. We are adoptive-parent gold dust.

I feel hot and dizzy. I look around the room at these children and babies, who all deserve a safe and loving home, and parents who will provide that and love them for ever. But despite the bright lights and sunshine streaming through the giant windows, despite the cheerful clothes of the children, there's a darkness in this room – in this situation – that creeps over my body. It feels so wrong, all of it. I understand that social workers have an impossible task, not least more than 5,000 children waiting in care for families they deserve. There are nowhere near enough approved families for these children, especially families who can reflect the children's different religious and cultural backgrounds. But we will not be finding our child this way. We run away, as fast as possible – a privilege these children do not have.

I find Amanda at breaktime the following week. She has already heard that the baby will have her name, and she's beaming. 'It's an honour being a nurse,' she tells me. 'Isn't it?'

I'm in awe of her. I tell her I'm glad she was there to save two lives at once. Maybe both mother and baby are alive because of her. I ask about military nursing and how it translates to 'normal' NHS nursing.

Amanda shakes her head. 'Both are about the team. Everything is about teamwork, that's what the military teaches you. And that's what the NHS teaches you.' She tells me that the most important aspect of military nursing is being non-judgemental. 'Nurses do not take sides,' she says. 'Everyone suffers in war – everyone. And the only thing that really helps, the only people who really understand, are those who stand beside you.' Then, in that instance, she looks far away in another place and time. I recognise that look.

I am working for a charity while doing my MA, caring for people in the community. I am there to nurse, but I rarely do any nursing tasks. One day I turn up to a small, stiflingly hot flat in Milton Keynes to care for an eight-year-old with a complex medical history and a life-limiting disease. Mohamed, the father, opens the door. He ushers me into a room where his wife crouches over a large, brightly coloured plastic bowl. She is making pickles. I offer to go and check on their daughter, but Mohamed tells me she's sleeping. Instead he takes my bag and gestures to the other side of the bucket, opposite his wife.

She speaks no English. But she does teach me how to make pickles. Mohamed likes to talk. He tells me of the dates he likes to eat, of the mountains, and the warmth of people in his home country. Then his experiences of being tortured there. And he looks far away, haunted. I think of my colleague, one of the best doctors I've ever worked with, from the same part of the world. How kind he is, as well as academic – he spends his time trying to translate what he calls 'hard science' into a language that I understand, showing me data graphs and numbers and symbols; and he laughs when I comment that I'm more of an artist than a scientist, and reminds me that medicine and nursing are both things in equal measure. How he brings the nurses hot food in small metal pots that he has cooked at home, as he thinks sandwiches are poison.

Mohamed lifts his shirt and turns to reveal a patterned back, much like the pattern on the plastic bowl. He tells of horrific events, but without sentiment. He simply wants me to know what happened; how he came to be in Britain. He does not cry or look sad. A nurse is a witness. We watch everything and we listen.

Nursing is complex and academic. It involves actions that appear simple from the outside, but are incredibly difficult. A nurse simply holding a patient's hand, for example, is assessing skin temperature, and turgor – elasticity – and signs of dehydration, and pulse, and respiratory rate and the emotional state of the patient. She is assessing the level of confusion, looking for signs of dementia, or acute kidney injury, or sepsis. While holding a patient's hand a nurse is assessing every aspect of a life: mental, emotional, psychological and physical health. She is trying to piece together the life in a snapshot, to understand what the person needs and how best to deliver it. Listening is like that, too. Active listening. Simple yet powerful, and crucial to delivering good nursing care. And so important for the patient. We all deserve to be heard.

I listen. I make pickles. Mohamed tells me about their health visitor who, he says, is also their friend. Health visitors are registered nurses with specialist qualifications, working across the NHS and beyond as public health practitioners. Health visitors work with babies and children up to five years old, or up to adulthood with at-risk or deprived groups such as those with disabilities, the homeless, addicts or travelling communities. 'We are lucky to have her,' he tells me.

I go into the bedroom to find a smiling girl with a feeding tube hooked up to an empty plastic pouch of milk, wearing earphones and watching a Disney film on a small TV. I wave and she waves back, then immediately returns to her film. She's used to nurses coming in and out. I disconnect her feed and head back to the parents and offer to stay and give them a break. I have spent hours with the parents, listening to Mohamed and making pickles, and only two minutes with my patient. But I'm coming to realise that you can't simply care for a patient as if they are somehow separate from a wider system. Caring for families is the (often unique) job of all nurses. Mohamed and his wife hug me, both of them, and usher me out.

Later, I find a plastic pot full of pickles in my bag and a note Sellotaped to it: *Thank you, Nurse. Come and see us again. You are always welcome in our home.*

Eamonn is the chief nurse at the Royal Marsden Hospital, the world's first specialist cancer hospital. He invites me into his office, and shows me the original letter written by Florence Nightingale on his wall. I am visiting to hear his thoughts about the importance of nursing. He tells me of the teams he's been a part of, and led, and how hard his colleagues work, their expertise and dedication to caring for patients and families going through cancer.

He is also a defence nurse and he has spent time saving lives in Iraq as well as in other field hospitals. I ask him about this military nursing, why he does it: risks his life, risks his mental health, sacrifices time with his family. I nod at the happy photo on his desk of his beautiful young family.

He becomes a tiny bit tearful. Then lifts his head, proudly. 'I do it for my colleagues,' he says without any hesitation whatsoever. 'These men and women who teach me the meaning of the word "teamwork".'

At the bus stop on the way home a nurse chats to me. She asks if I'm visiting and on discovering I'm a nurse too, here to interview Eamonn, she puts her hand on her chest, over her heart. 'He's a brilliant leader,' she says. 'The kindest person. He has helped me through some really hard days. Always speaks up for us nurses.'

A few months later, and we have suddenly been plunged into a new reality: COVID-19 sweeping through and permanently changing our world in a matter of weeks. I am deciding whether to join the nursing register once more, even for a short time, on the newly formed COVID-19 emergency register. I am afraid. I think of my family, my children, my choices. And then I see a photo of one of the new NHS Nightingale

Hospitals and the nurses who will be at the helm. There Eamonn stands in front, head held high, in his nurse's uniform. He will be the chief nurse.

I think of how fragile he is. And how strong. I think of teamwork, and the importance of it in every single hospital and community and social-care setting, by nurses, doctors, carers, cooks, delivery drivers, porters, physiotherapists, mental-health support workers, cleaners and so many more. They are not heroes. Just ordinary people doing their jobs. But there is plenty of courage. I think of my patients over the years, of their families, their bravery. I think of my colleagues who keep health and social care running even now, and of all the human ingredients that make up the NHS. I am frightened. But still, I want to stand alongside my colleagues. I fill in the registration form.

5

Decorated Veterans

The day my daughter is called the N-word starts out like any other. It is May and sunny and lovely, and we've come in the early evening to the local park with a ball to kick around. She's learning to run, always falling and grazing her knees, so we spend a lot of time in the park; grass is the safest option. And it's her favourite place. She isn't yet talking – just gobbledegook, a language that only I can understand. But she already dances, twirling and doing roly-polys and jumping and spinning. I watch her run away and then run back, giggling with delight as she comes towards me, never tiring of stretching her arms out so that I can lift her and swing her around. Life could not be more perfect.

I don't hear the words at first. I can see a group of four young men on the other side of the park, looking in our direction. They're standing with their tops off, drinking cans of beer, and a short, thick-necked dog runs between them.

I am used to people looking at my daughter. She is so beautiful that people stop all the time to look at her, so I don't pay the group of men much attention. I can hear the sound of an ice-cream van in the distance, so at first it's hard to notice the shouting. I let my face travel upwards towards the sunshine and close my eyes, breathing in the smell of a far-away first seasonal barbecue. And then I hear it. That word. The ice-cream van stops, and my daughter runs away again, giggling. I hear more words, shouted in our direction: N-lover, N, Coon.

My heart thumps so loudly I can no longer hear the words, but as I open my eyes I can see at once that my baby daughter has heard them. She stops laughing and is standing perfectly still, looking at the men who are shouting straight at her. One of them throws a can in her direction. He yells something as he throws it. The dog barks and barks. I watch her step backwards as though the can has hit her; confused and terrified tears fall down her face, although she does not make a sound. She runs towards me, but for the first time she doesn't stretch out her arms. I haven't protected her. My arms around her are useless.

In that second I realise my daughter will experience a different world from mine. A hateful and dangerous world. My white privilege means I'll never truly understand how racism feels, not in the way my children will, that my partner does. I still have so much work to do. I need to keep listening, and learning, from both my partner and many, many others. I need to understand – and fight – the structural racism that has benefited me and all white people.

Another adoption preparation day. Today there's a giant bucket of KFC chicken on the middle table, as the M&S sandwiches have not arrived in time for our scheduled lunch break. A significant proportion of the prospective adopters are unable to eat the non-halal chicken. A broken clock clicks every five seconds or so and shows the time: 2.10. It is hot in the room and smells of greasy food. Teniola is today wearing jeans tucked into her cowboy boots, and has spoken for much of the morning about the importance of co-sleeping to promote attachment. But she moves on to race, and culture and identity and belonging. 'Placements where adopted parents have a different cultural and racial background from their child have a particularly high disruption rate,' she says.

I notice her careful use of the word 'disruption' instead of 'failure'; 'child' instead of 'baby'. Everyone wants a baby.

'It's important you can anticipate trans-racial and trans-cultural challenges that might be experienced by your child.'

We are planning to adopt a child from a mixed-heritage background, like ours, so we reflect their background as much as possible. But my heart speeds up and I begin to panic. I think about that day in the park; and another day when we find that someone has lined up fascist leaflets from our front door all the way to my daughter's nursery, and we walk our route, picking them up like the breadcrumbs in 'Hansel and Gretel'. Except that these breadcrumbs say: *Go Home. Back to where you came from.* The police are kind, but unable to reassure us they will find whoever did these things, let alone be able to charge them. I need to really think about how I support my mixed-heritage children with the racism they will surely face.

After lunch Teniola moves on to discuss all the potential reasons children might end up in the care system. In the vast majority of cases, she tells us, families keep their birth children, with support, even if the parents have drug and alcohol addictions, severe mental illness or significant learning disabilities – or all of those things combined. She talks of the extremes. She talks about mental-health disorders that are so severe there is no way a birth family will be able to keep a child safe. 'It's hard for me to explain how some serious mental illnesses can affect people's lives,' she says. But I can imagine.

I am with the community mental-health team, and they have warned me about the house we are going to visit. The pathway is full of rubbish: large bags of papers, a supermarket trolley, two broken fridges, a fractured garden gnome, weeds everywhere. We knock on the door. Nobody answers. The nurse I am working with – Aditi – reaches underneath the doormat for a key. 'He can't get to the door,' she tells me. She's carrying a bag full of documentation and drugs, but also a rape alarm. Community nursing is sometimes a dangerous business. The team tries to allocate two nurses for some clients and certain estates, but it's not always possible, and a lone nurse is always at greater risk of assault. Aditi is slight, an ex-dancer. She retrained as a mental health nurse after a serious leg injury. 'I always wanted to work with mental health,' she says. 'I had a total breakdown after my injury: physical and mental. And the mental health nurses gave me back my life.'

Aditi opens the door and shouts as she does so, 'Mr George. It's the nurses come to see how you are.'

I recall my first-ever trip abroad so vividly at this moment. We went to Tunisia, and I was ten; the aeroplane door opened and the heat and smell burst in, almost knocking me over. Mr George's hallway has the same effect on me. I stagger backwards. The smell of his house quite literally makes my eyes water and my throat burn. I have to lean forward and rest my hands on my thighs and take deep breaths. Aditi does the same. We look at one another and venture in.

The hallway is stacked, floor to ceiling, with newspapers. There is a thin path through and, luckily, we are both small enough to fit. We head into the smell, as though into a sewer, and towards the living room at the end of the corridor. I fully expect to find Mr George dead, flies buzzing around him. But the television is on and a voice shouts out, 'Hello?'

He is sitting in a high-backed chair, the kind you get in care homes, with a plastic coating and wooden arms. But it takes me a while to see a human being. The room is entirely full of junk. It looks like the inside of a skip. Mr George himself is sitting camouflaged among hundreds of newspapers. Aditi opens a window. 'How have you been?'

He moves and the newspapers rustle. 'Not too bad.'

On a table next to him there is a pile of coins, an old train ticket, a *Radio Times*, a pill dispenser, a glass of water and an overflowing ashtray. Mr George is smoking a cigarette but there is another, still lit, in the ashtray. There's no evidence of smoke alarms, and so many newspapers and magazines are piled up and around Mr George and all over the room. On the mantelpiece a pile of bills teeters next to an old record player covered in a thick layer of dust. There are photographs everywhere, old ones, most of them black and white, of a young and handsome Mr George and a woman who I assume is – or was – his wife. He sees me looking at them, and his eyes slowly follow mine to a large photo on the wall. In it Mr George is impossibly handsome and cheerful, wearing a military uniform and holding the waist of a woman, who is smiling and beautiful. Comparing him now to the man in the photo is at once heartbreaking and terrifying. I know that he has a diagnosis of depression. But he is the saddest-looking human being I have ever seen.

Aditi does so many things at once. She risk-assesses him. She makes numerous phone calls to the various networks of people who look after him, the urgent-care team and a cleaning company that specialises in people who are not well. They understand that things need to be done gradually and bit by bit. 'People who hoard can die, if things are cleaned suddenly overnight,' Aditi tells me later.

There's no talk of him moving to hospital. She puts in place daily carers, administers his medication and documents his care plan. Mr George simply stares at the television throughout it all, almost catatonic. I try and chat to him, ask him about the photos, but he seems to find it hard to talk, as though he doesn't have the energy to open his mouth. But he does follow me around the room with his eyes. I can tell he is listening. I help move the newspapers from under his chair and discover a box of medals beneath them. I put them next to him, on the table, and ask him about them, but he merely shrugs. I wonder why he got them, how brave he must have been, how many lives he might have saved – or taken.

I help Aditi wash Mr George, peeling the newspapers away where they have stuck to his sweaty skin, and try and wash the headlines that have transferred, like tattoos, to his arms. He continues to stare straight ahead.

'Do you think about harming yourself?' Aditi asks him.

He slowly moves his head to look at her. Then shakes it. It's clear that he is too sad even to hurt himself. It's as though he is not really in this world. He is a shell. A shadow. Depression is an infinitely cruel disease.

Nursing teaches you that there is always something worse. Martin is admitted to the acute psychiatric ward after he drops his trousers on the top deck of the number 203 bus and, while masturbating, shouts that he is the son of Jesus and is there to spread the seed of God around the world. The bus driver, who has seen it all before, is 'not having it' and throws Martin off the bus, leaving him distressed and vulnerable – one shoe on, one shoe off – at the roadside outside Luton's Arndale shopping centre, still shouting about the Messiah and the coming of new gods. People simply walk on by. But then he drops his trousers again and the police are called when, according to Stephen, a deadpan – and sometimes cruel – nursing assistant, Martin 'tries to fire his penis off like a machine gun to a crowd of schoolchildren'. He tells the police that he is giving them the chance of everlasting life and redemption with his magic seed, and is sectioned under the Mental Health Act, being considered a danger both to himself and to other people.

Despite how seriously ill Martin is, I learn that he could get better quickly with the right treatments, and although it's hard for me to imagine this, I already know there are many surprises in mental-health nursing. I've seen people who are catatonic, unable to walk, talk, wash or feed themselves, be back eating meals in the dining room within days, chatting about *Coronation Street*. One of my patients – or service users – a veterinary nurse, is convinced that an alien abduction has taken place. She believes her C-section scars are from the lasers that the aliens used when replacing her internal organs with a planet, which will eventually grow so large that she will burst open and a new universe will explode from her; and that this is how our present universe was created, too. She tried to reopen the scars in order to dig out this growing planet before it became too big, and was found operating on her own abdomen with a cat-spaying kit. She is home within weeks and back at work, helping to spay cats again, shortly after that.

There are other people who do not recover. I find the most upsetting aspect of mental-health nursing those who somehow, despite the best care, medication, therapy and nurses, never seem to get better and roll between services like a slow, sad snooker ball. There are frequent visitors to the mental-health services, just as there are to A&E; often they are the same visitors. Mental health nurses are experts at getting to the core of such people. But medication sometimes only treats the surface – if anything at all. For some people it is important and often lifesaving, and for others, a senior mental health nurse tells me, it can be harmful. 'Anything deeper requires a close, careful look at the person's whole life and history, and such therapy is expensive and takes time. Time and money that the NHS does not have.'

Martin is extremely unwell when we first meet. He has no insight into his condition, which the nurse in charge says is a blessing, because up until the point of admission he'd been living a fairly ordinary life. He was training to be a mechanic, with a full apprenticeship, and was doing very well at the local further-education college. He had friends, many of them from school, with whom he smoked a lot of skunk. But one day he simply could not get out of bed. He'd had an epiphany – a dream or a vision. During the night an angel, whom Martin describes as 'wearing a white gown and glowing with light', told him that he is the new Messiah. That the survival of the human race depends on him. And the only way he can save the world is with his seed. Martin dismissed the hallucination and stopped smoking skunk. But increasingly, over the following weeks and months, he heard the voice of the angel inside his head. And he began to believe that his sperm is the only thing that can save humankind. At first he collected it in a pot, wiping it on walls and playground equipment. But the voice told him that the healing comes from him, and that his seed loses potency almost as soon as it's outside his body. Matters escalated.

Martin shows me a notebook where he has written everything the angel says to him. It's alarming: full of biro scrawls of eyes and teeth, the writing as scratched and sharp as if written with a compass instead of a pen. He's scratched through the pages in places, and there are small tears in the paper. The pen changes to pencil (he is only allowed a blunt pencil, because he is deemed at risk of harm from using pens), but the words, although less sharp and spiky, are increasingly incoherent:

You are the saviour. Your seed is the name of God and the only way to save the masses is to protect them with the seed of God. The dark angel is casting a shadow over the world and the end is coming and you twbbbbb odkhtt sfjkyhpf SSSSEEEEEEDDDDDDDDDDDD God JESUS kill. KILLLLLL. The SEEDD savingsaving. Thhhhhhhhhoddd children, all the children.

'I am the son of Jesus,' Martin tells me. 'And inside me is all the light of the universe. The Apocalypse is coming for all of us and, when it does, only those chosen will survive. A new age will begin.'

I have been allocated Martin and three other people to look after: all suffering from major depression. But it is Martin who is taking up most of my time. I can see that he is looking for clues as to whether or not I believe him, or if I am in fact working for MI6, which he thinks is trying to prevent him from saving the world. I try to keep my face neutral. But I yawn by accident. 'I'm so sorry,' I say.

Martin frowns. 'You're tired of me,' he says.

'Oh no. No, I'm so sorry. I'm just tired. I had a late night.'

'Sleep is the first symptom of the disease spreading,' he says. 'Nobody will sleep. Then all the food will be contaminated, and then the rivers and the seas and the mountains. We will one by one die in pain.' He is manic, I can see, and I'm not sure what to say or do. He begins to pace up and down the corridor, caged, dangerous, desperate. I decide the best thing to do is give him some space, and maybe my absence and his pacing will help him relax a bit. But, really, I have no idea how to help him.

I do some checks on the others. One of them is on fifteen-minute checks. Sometimes nurses cannot leave a person at all, and I've often wondered how hard that must be in terms of dignity: to have someone staring at you all the time, even while you use the bathroom. But of course it may be necessary to keep people alive. Keeping people safe, until they can keep themselves safe, a kind of supportive critical care for the mind.

When I get back to Martin, he's sitting in the room where people are encouraged to do art or music or creative writing, and he's reading a book upside down. 'Do you want to turn it around, Martin?' I gesture to the upside-down book on his lap.

'Are you mad?' he says. He taps the book. 'That's how they know.'

He has started repeatedly flicking his head in an odd movement to one side. This tic could be a nasty side-effect of his medication.

'Would you like some tea or coffee?'

He shakes his head vigorously. 'I don't drink caffeine,' he says. 'It is a drug, you know.'

I think of all the drugs he's taking – the concoction that's hit-and-miss until they get it right, or not. I think of his smoking skunk and how he told me he started smoking at eleven years old. I learn that Martin is vegetarian and doesn't drink alcohol or caffeine.

'I've got this cat called Bertie,' he says, beaming.

'Is someone caring for Bertie while you're in hospital?'

'My neighbour has a key. She said she'd give him food.'

I'm relieved. It's not unheard of for pets to be forgotten, if someone gets admitted suddenly. Often animals are family members and it can cause such distress that their pets are not being cared for that I've known nurses go and feed cats. Once a nurse even took a patient's dog home, after the patient in question suffered a stroke. She used to bring the dog to the stroke rehabilitation unit occasionally, to reunite them.

Martin puts his book down, and his face changes. He looks at his hands, his arms, and I see a flash of shock in his eyes as if he has remembered something really important. They fill with tears and he looks at me.

'How did I get here? There were police – I remember police.' And he rocks back and forth, back and forth, trying to remember.

I am too scared to say anything, in case I say something wrong. Martin will now be on a sex-offender list for ever. He will get better and will only then understand the things he did when he was extremely unwell. The things he had no control over. Actions that may well define the rest of his life.

Maybe he is remembering already. I stand opposite him and try and think of something helpful to say. But I can't.

Martin looks at me in horror, and I see in his eyes that he has insight. He is getting better and he is remembering.

I found caring for Mr George the saddest thing. But despite making judgements about Martin – and his behaviour and illness – before I knew him, I must turn my head away before I start to cry. I have never seen a man more broken.

Mental health nurses and the communities they work with understand uncertainty. They know that any one of us could become as sick as Mr George or Martin. It could happen to me. Or to you. I'm struggling to cope with that knowledge. I'm questioning my ability to be a nurse or find any pleasure at all in the job, in the muddiness of it, the many shades of grey. The qualified nurses are so professional, proficient and fluid. They are philosophical about everything, and so kind they must ache. I wonder if I should quit nursing altogether: the sadness is too much. But I find my smile again, my laugh.

As a student nurse on the unit, today my job is to fill in admission paperwork. I'm relieved. My first patient is Ava, who was ill as a child, but with the right support and therapy got better. It wasn't until she was studying law that she became seriously ill again, and was diagnosed with a personality disorder as well as depression and generalised anxiety disorder. It's hard to imagine so many labels attached to such a young person, just a few months younger than I am. I wonder if they will be helpful or not. I imagine them attached to me, how they might feel stuck onto my skin. I roll the word 'disorder' around in my head, and hear an echo: chaos. I, too, am chaotic. What young person isn't?

There are a ton of questions, and Ava is too sick to answer any of them. Her face is tired, sad and confused. She has been started on medication, which makes her mouth very, very dry, and I notice her cracked, almost bleeding lips. I feel so sorry for her. Ava is quiet and nearly invisible on the ward. She does not interact with the other patients or staff. She keeps her eyes to the ground the whole time, and I don't hear her voice except in whispers. But after lunch there is shouting. And then laughing. Loud, almost hysterical laughing bursts through the ward. I make out Ava's voice. Then I see her pointing to something on the ground. A cleaner screams, running past. 'There's a rat, a rat!'

I jump back involuntarily, and then stop. Ava is cry-laughing holding her sides. She is pointing to a rat, very still, squished against the skirting board. I have no idea why she is laughing.

Laif, a serious and well meaning psychiatrist, is walking towards us, hand over his mouth, totally bald. He usually has hair. I look down at the 'rat' and realise it's not a rat at all.

We never find out how Laif's toupee fell off, or if it was pulled off, or how it ended up in the corridor. He doesn't mention it. Instead he bends down, snatches it up and walks into the staff office, bald head held high.

'It came off,' says Ava, screeching with laughter. 'It was a wig.'

And I stare straight at her, make my stomach hard as she laughs and laughs. I have never wanted to laugh more.

I have always had an awful habit of laughing at the wrong moment. Bursting out into uncontrolled cackling at entirely inappropriate times. I know where I get that trait. After my dad dies, a funeral director comes to the house to go through things with my mum, my brother and me. He is exactly as I'd imagined a funeral director: sombre, respectful, wearing a clean dark suit with polished black shoes, which he takes off at the door. My mum sits next to my brother on the couch and I sit opposite the funeral director, as he discusses viewing my dad's body, the different types of casket, the possibility of cremation. Unfortunately his voice is funny: high and low, as if singing. My mum is the first to burst out laughing, and my brother follows soon afterwards. They bury their faces in each other's shoulders, crying with laughter at every word the man says. I try to keep a straight face: it is only a matter of days since my dad died, and we are raw with grief. But it is funny – so funny. Somehow I hold it in, although the walls ring with the sound of my dad, who would have been holding his stomach and laughing, too. I try to apologise and make out that my family are sobbing, not laughing, giving the firmest eye contact I can manage, in order to distract the funeral director from my brother and mum rolling around on the couch.

Later we have a group ward round to which Ava is invited, as is standard. I have the task of listening and recording everything that is said in a large black diary. I am the scribe – the term we give the nurse who is writing down information in real time. We are in the staffroom on the mental-health ward, with a *Confidential meeting in progress* sign Sellotaped to the door's window, and all of us sitting on scratchy wool-covered chairs. I still feel a fizzing in the back of my throat from holding in laughter earlier. I swallow it away. Laif has replaced his toupee. Ava is quiet once more. I write each considered question from Laif and the team about whether Ava understands the side-effects of her medication, or whether she is feeling any other symptoms of illness. I am ready to write down each answer carefully in perfect handwriting. But then I look up. First I notice Ava pressing her mouth closed as if she's holding something in. Then I follow her eyes. Laif's hurriedly re-attached toupee has slipped to one side. He nods, and it moves a fraction more.

The room gets hotter and hotter with each question and subsequent nod of encouragement from Laif.

'How long have you been feeling like this?'

'Do you know where you are?'

'Ava, we'd like to talk this through but you need to engage if you can. I know this is difficult but try and talk to us.'

Ava presses her lips together even harder. She puts her hands palm down on the table and leans on them. Laif's toupee is dangerously close to falling off.

I hold in the laughter once more until it hurts, press my feet down hard on the ground as Ava presses her hands on the table.

I can see it all. Her chaos and her humour. And she looks straight at me and I know that she can see the same in me. There is a huge power imbalance in the room, and the situation is horrific. Ava should be having fun with her friends, starting her adult life with adventures and love and hope and freedom. Instead she is stuck in hospital, seriously ill. But when she eventually opens her mouth it's laughter that spills out of her, and, for a few moments, whether it is right to laugh at someone's appearance or not, I can't help but find beauty in the sound of it.

Laif leans forwards and his toupee reaches his eyebrows. But Ava is not watching him. Instead she is staring right at me. A single tear of laughter travels down my cheek. Ava watches me as she laughs, and she can see how desperate I am to join in with her. Laif looks from Ava to me then back again, confused as to what we are clearly finding funny. We concentrate on each other, two young women, and, finally, I can no longer hold it in.

6

A Hamster Named Batman

My daughter is having a spectacular tantrum. In the same way that a sick child will somehow suppress their symptoms at a GP's appointment and perk up into perfect health, so my usually well-behaved daughter turns into the devil-child as soon as our social worker rings the doorbell. She is holding her breath and thumping the ground with her fists when Deepa comes in, and then my daughter gasps, bangs her head on the floor and screams.

'Having fun?' Deepa tries to put us at ease, but there's nothing easy about this.

I smile too brightly and flash a look to my daughter that says, *For God's sake, stop screaming,* which surely Deepa notices.

I kneel down on the ground and gently stroke my daughter's back, despite the look I gave her, and hum a song that I know she likes. She loves singing. She loves music, but instead of nursery rhymes she prefers rock. She dances and plays air-guitar for hours to the Rolling Stones, Kings of Leon and Guns N' Roses. She only tolerates me humming a lullaby. For a second she calms a bit, her breathing slows down and I think I have won. But she is whip-smart, even at three, and she can smell my anxiety, sense my will and absorb the atmosphere in a room through her skin. All children can do this with their mothers. Clever things.

She hits me on the arm and, even though she is still pretty much preverbal, she clearly shouts, 'Bugger' at the top of her voice.

And despite my very best efforts to maintain composure and calm, her frustration and screaming rush through me and ignite something, and I cannot hide my anger as I say through gritted teeth, 'Stop this right now.' And I pick my daughter up and carry her out of the room. I am seeing red. I sit her on the stairs, which have long been her 'naughty step', and I try and breathe. 'You will stay here and think about your behaviour for three whole minutes.' And then I go back to Deepa, still shaking.

'I'm so sorry. I'm so sorry. I don't know why she's being like this.'

But Deepa can barely hear me, as my daughter is howling like a wolf. She stops, briefly, and despite her poor verbal skills she then begins to sing her favourite song by Kings of Leon: 'Sex on Fire'.

The home study is the part of the adoption process when the social worker allocated to you visits over a number of months to examine every single aspect of your life. It is incredibly stressful, for everything rests on what kind of assessment she or he makes. Nor is it limited to the prospective adopters.

Deepa plans to speak to everyone in our lives, from our ex-partners, to individual chats alone with our existing children, to referees, employers, banks. There is no hiding from this process. As with therapy, our darkest secrets will be exposed, discussed and assessed. Deepa keeps reassuring me that they are not looking for perfect parents, because such a thing does not exist. But she also keeps saying that they need to be confident that we can parent therapeutically, because all adopted children have special needs in one form or another, even if they are adopted from birth: 'Children with additional needs require extra-resilient parents.'

I keep thinking of the 20 per cent of children who, I'm told, end up back in care; whose adoptive parents couldn't cope, even if they had the best intentions, because the damage was too great. 'You never know how trauma will manifest itself in a child. And there is no greater trauma than losing a birth mother. None at all in the world.' I nod. But I disagree. I think of all the mothers and families of sick children that I have ever cared for. The enormity of their grief, if the child doesn't make it. This is the most unspeakable, unthinkable thing of all. There is no greater tragedy in the world than losing a child. I picture my nan, and the photograph of her son next to her bed. The last photo of him before he died, aged four. Underneath the photo is a poem. I'm not sure where it's from, but I've always loved it:

God has taken back our darling,
Placed our bud amongst his flowers,
Taken back the child he lent us
To a better place than ours.

I know my nan has never, ever recovered from losing a child and it left a giant hole in the heart of our family, for ever. She is an elderly woman now and not a day goes by when she doesn't miss him until it hurts.

I try to stop thinking of it and focus instead on the joyful possibility of a new child to love. But I can't stop thinking about birth mothers and the pain they must feel on losing a child, on having a child taken, whatever the circumstances. I try and switch it off, close it down. But it sits, and settles, somewhere under my ribs. And I wake at night, heart-angry, mouth-dry, and think of how adoption trauma is impossible for a child to recover from. I know what that looks like. I've seen it at work. And I've heard about it, especially from my mum.

My mum, who taught me the language of kindness, begins her training to be a child-protection social worker at the time I am a wayward teen in full swing. I am caught up in hanging around parks with my friends, smoking and drinking Mad Dog 20/20 and generally being the kind of teen who could probably do with a social worker herself. That my mum wants to work with babies and children and teenagers doesn't surprise me. She is soft and gentle and full of love, and she has been a nursery nurse for many years, always surrounded by children. But I've never imagined her as tough, or having the kind of grit that surely child-protection social workers must need. When she qualifies and begins working long days, duty weekends and some nights, I sense a shift in her. She is tired, which is understandable, but there is something more than that – deeper. She looks haunted. She stops sleeping.

It is years later that she explains her lack of sleep to me, and later still that I begin to try and understand all that she has witnessed. But I'll never really understand. Not really. Social work, like nursing, is the kind of job that is near-impossible to imagine from the outside. How many times must my mum have known that children were in unsafe situations, yet due to a lack of resources could do nothing at all about it. How many times must she have done a routine visit to a household and have walked out, carrying a baby so badly abused or neglected there was simply nothing else to do, despite having nowhere else to place the baby. How many birth mothers must my mum have empathised with and desperately tried to help keep their children safe, so that she did not have to take them into care.

She doesn't ever give details about her work. But I understand that haunted look she has, and I admire the fact that – despite the things she must have seen, and had to do – she continues to do the job, with little thanks or reward. Because, as she always says, children are the most important people of all. And I realise just how much grit she has. She is the kindest, strongest person I know. We talk every possibility through. I want to go into adoption with my eyes wide open. It is my mum who listens to my worries about the trauma of adoption, then reminds me of the most important thing: the trauma of staying in a family that cannot keep a child safe is far, far worse.

The children's oncology day unit is decorated in a way that is trying to be as cheerful as possible: tropical birds are painted on the walls, at child's-eye level, alongside elephants and giraffes, and a buffalo that looks more like a cow and a bit out of place. There's a television showing a cartoon, and a play area with toys and books being chewed on by a toddler, who is wearing a miniature hospital gown and appears to be able to move only one side of his body. A woman – perhaps his mum – sits on a plastic chair, looking out of the window.

I follow Polly into the treatment room. Polly is quick. I am always impressed by how calm and upbeat she seems to be – this despite working exclusively in paediatric oncology. But she's not smiling today. Biting her lip, she is close to tears and wringing her hands anxiously. The treatment room looks much like a GP's clinic: a thin bed, an even thinner pair of curtains, a sideboard with stackable plastic containers holding different cannula, blood bottles, steri-strips, gauze squares and alcowipes.

A teenage girl is propped up on the bed and has a thick red cut on her neck. She is clearly agitated, swearing at the doctor who is sitting beside her, holding her arm. She has a Hickman line in her chest, a thick line that delivers chemo-therapy drugs. She is thin and covered in bruises.

'This is India,' Polly tells me. 'She was admitted with AML and has been tying ligatures around her neck. Her foster carer is en route.'

Acute Myeloid Leukaemia is a cancer of the white blood cells. White blood cells help to fight infection and normally these cells, which are produced in the bone marrow, repair and reproduce themselves in an orderly and controlled way. In leukaemia, however, the process gets out of control and the cells continue to divide, but do not mature. It is the only cancer that is more common in children than in adults. But it's not the cancer that has led to the crash call for India.

'Hi, India.' I sit down on the other side of her, and the doctor lets go of her arm. 'I'm Christie. I'm one of the nurses.'

She begins to swear. I put my arm around her, but she jolts backwards.

The doctor – a woman I do not recognise – stands up. 'I'll be over there,' she says. She nods to the nurses' station, where there are a few computers. 'But she needs admitting. We're just not sure where.'

'I don't want to move anywhere,' India shouts. She turns to me. 'I want to go home.'

'Well, it looks as if your foster carer is on her way in,' I say. 'I don't think you'll be able to go home today, but when she gets here, Polly will chat to you both, I'm sure, and make a plan. Clearly you're not feeling great.' I gesture to the ligature mark.

I can already see that she doesn't need intensive care. She is conscious and speaking, and alert and not confused. The quality of her voice tells me that she has a clear and functioning airway, and her respiratory rate is within normal limits. But she needs one-to-one nursing, and sending her home would not be safe. She requires a nurse who is trained in mental and physical health in equal measures. Like all of us do.

'Do you know about me?' she asks.

I shake my head. 'Only what Polly told me.'

'I tied a belt around my neck,' she says. She points to the red line. And out of nowhere she screams and bangs the back of her head on the wall. 'I just want to die.'

A bump appears almost immediately. I call out for help. I try and hold India, but she's shrugging me off, and she's pulling and biting at her Hickman line.

I shout louder and pull the crash bell again.

Her Hickman line goes straight into a major blood vessel and, if she bites through it, she could bleed to death. 'Stop it, India,' I say. 'Help!' I call out again.

Polly rushes back in, wearing an apron, closely followed by another nurse. They take her arms – India is so weak she cannot stop them – and sit by her side until her breathing slows down.

'Clearly,' Polly says later, away from India, 'she needs one-to-one care. Psychiatric intensive care. The problem we have is that the mental health ward won't accept a child having chemo, and the high-dependency unit is not equipped for a child with mental-health issues. We need to get a mental health nurse to special her on HDU, alongside a paediatric nurse. Or something. We've tried all agencies and there's no one. There's no bed for hundreds of miles and, even then, not for seventy-two hours at least. What am I supposed to do?'

'Sorry for being such a problem,' India shouts, 'by having cancer.' She's shouting louder and louder. A small, bald girl pushing a drip-stand walks by. Her nurse hurries her up. But as the girl walks past, she turns her head, very slowly, her eyes wide and frightened. I am not surprised. I feel frightened, too. It's hard even to look at India. Her body is a map of hurt: she has scars and cuts and bruises, and now she has a huge bump on her head. But it's the hurt on her face, behind her eyes, that is much more painful to witness.

India's foster carer is a woman named Evelyn, who says she has 'two others she needs to get back to' and tells the hospital social worker that she can't cope with India any more. 'She's spent her whole life in and out of different settings:

other foster carers, residential homes, mental-health wards. She even went back to the birth family for a few months, and that's when things got really bad.'

She seems tired and her face is hard. She's seen too much.

'Some children you can't help,' she goes on. 'Children's mental illness is the plague of our times. But because we can't see it or catch it, we can pretend it's not there.'

I learn that India was eating her own vomit when the social workers found her at the age of two. Her parents had been using heroin and there was violence, and eventually the flat became a place where drug addicts were in and out, and more than likely there was sexual, physical and emotional abuse as well as neglect. 'She tried to burn my house down,' Evelyn says, shrugging, 'when she first came to me at twelve. She'd had a failed adoption and had been through four other foster families before that. It was me or a residential home. Last-chance saloon.'

'You kept her? After that? Do you not worry she'll do it again?'

Evelyn shrugs again, but looks over at India. 'We go from one thing to the next. I doubt she'll do that again. She likes to surprise me.'

I watch her watching India. And I realise that Evelyn loves her. As hard as it is to love her, she does. 'I don't know how you do it,' I say, honestly. 'And then the leukaemia. It's too cruel. Unbelievable.'

But Evelyn snorts. 'Leukaemia is the least of her worries,' she says. And I know she means it. 'In the scheme of her life, cancer is a road bump. When you have sawn off your arm, you forget your cancer, for a while at least.'

I had Evelyn so wrong at first – thinking she was a bit indifferent to India. But I can see that she is wise and loving, and tough at the same time. The kind of mum that India needs.

'Do you think she'll ever be adopted again?'

'No chance. Some children in the care system are simply unable to live in families. The problem is that until they've tried to live in a family, you don't know that.'

'Nobody can help me,' India says. And she doesn't cry, but looks at me with such misery that I have to stop myself from crying.

'You ready now?' Polly asks her.

India doesn't nod. But she doesn't shake her head, either. Maybe that's as good as it gets. Evelyn doesn't really try and comfort her, I notice, but when we get to the treatment room, she sits next to India as Polly cleans her Hickman line. They don't speak. But Evelyn pulls out some nail polish from her bag, and India stretches out her arm without looking at her.

One by one, Evelyn paints India's nails, until they are all midnight-blue. She does this with great concentration, in total silence. Then she blows on them. She blows on them for a long time after I suspect they are dry. Gently. Then she hums a song.

India looks directly up at Evelyn with her sad eyes, and there is a flicker of something beautiful between them. And I see determination on Evelyn's face. The courage to care.

Of course children can suffer terrible trauma and mental illness even when they have stable, caring and loving birth families. So many of them do, and the number of children and adolescents experiencing serious mental illness is ever-increasing. No parent can guarantee that their child won't experience trauma, or serious mental illness, or even lose their lives due to it. No matter how careful they are.

Olivia is just six years old when she stops eating breakfast. Her teachers at her primary school become concerned when she begins to faint regularly – she is referred to the school nurse, who manages a growing number of schools. They notice that Olivia is throwing away her sandwiches, and at break and lunchtimes she runs around, but not like the other children. Instead of playing with them, Olivia runs laps, even jogging on the spot if it is too busy for her to move at speed. Her parents are called into school, but aren't overly concerned – after all, what six-year-old doesn't run around and sometimes act in a picky way with food?

But Olivia's weight loss is dramatic. The school nurse tells the parents she'd like to refer Olivia to the CAMHS team: the Child and Adolescent Mental Health Services, who provide support for any child or adolescent who needs emotional or mental-health care. But Olivia's health deteriorates while her name sits on the long waiting list: her knees become the widest part of her legs, and she can easily get her fingers all the way round her upper arm. By the time she turns seven and is admitted to hospital as an emergency, she is seriously ill. Her head is disproportionate to her body and her skin is translucently pale, with blue-green veins snaking across her forehead. Her eyes are dull and, even though she is listless, she continues to move, marching on the spot, unable to keep still, her legs constantly moving. Olivia has begun to make herself sick when eating any food, and she drinks water in such vast quantities that her belly swells out underneath her concave chest. She looks to me like a starving child. She *is* a starving child.

The ward I'm currently on placement with has many children who have been referred by community CAMHS, identified as needing in-patient care to keep them safe – or even alive. Children are admitted with mental-health problems ranging from somatic or conversion disorders to psychosis and eating disorders that have made their daily life impossible. Olivia waited months for an assessment via CAMHS and is now too unwell to have talking or family therapy in the community.

She is brought to hospital in an ambulance, having suffered a seizure. She has a nasogastric tube inserted and is put on to bed rest, to conserve what little energy she has left. Her blood-sugar levels are dangerously low; the staff are worried she might have further seizures or even be at risk of falling into a coma, so she has a drip inserted and a glucose solution infused through a vein. Her heart rate is much too slow. I sit beside her and watch her neck vein pulsating, a steady but slow beat, her veins protruding so much, working so hard. Her face is covered in soft hair – lanugo, a sort of downy fuzz, sometimes seen on newborn babies, particularly if they are premature. In Olivia's case it is a response, a nurse tells me later, to the hypothermia that is ever-present in children with anorexia. 'Her body is trying to insulate itself, growing hair to keep out the cold.'

The ward is decorated in bright primary colours, with comfortable sofas and televisions, bedrooms decorated with photographs, quilt covers from home, soft toys and computer games. It is homely and welcoming, but it feels almost too calm, too quiet, a bit too clutter-free. There are no piles of laundry, or unopened mail or leftover cereal bowls, no muddy wellies by the door. Regardless, for the children who are staying in these seven in-patient beds, this environment is lifesaving. The nurses are lifesaving. They develop such close relationships with the children that they become family – surrogate parents for children who need to live away from home in order to get better. Visiting by parents is often limited to one or two evenings per week and to daytimes at the weekend, depending on the age of the child.

The nurses deliver family therapy, psycho-education, personalised holistic care that includes risk assessment, and innovative research projects that inform clinical guidelines. They deliver outreach education to nurses from non-specialised areas of the hospital who are caring for children with mental-health disorders or autism or learning disabilities. The most important role of the nurse, though, is to be with the patients. To spend time together, particularly at mealtimes, and to build functional and positive relationships. 'We encourage the parents to eat with us, too, on the evening they visit,' I am told. But the nurse doesn't expand on that. I wonder if the parents are being assessed, too – and why parents are encouraged only to visit one or two evenings a week, instead of every evening. I soon understand that it's families who need to be treated if a child is ill, or the child will never recover.

The nurses are part of the family therapy that her parents are encouraged to attend. I spend the day with the parents, getting to know Olivia and her family. Olivia has a face full of freckles. 'Angels' kisses,' she says and laughs, weakly. Her laugh is wet, as if she's an older person with heart failure. Of course her heart may well be damaged. Anorexia can cause a number of heart-related problems. It is the leading cause of mental-health deaths, either through the physical effects of the disease on the body's organs, or by suicide. It is desperately sad to see Olivia consumed by the illness. I watch her, still trying to keep moving; her downy hair, her concave chest, her muscle-wasted legs. It's as if her mind is slowly eating her body, cancelling her out bit by bit, shrinking her down and down until she doesn't exist. Perhaps when it's impossible to make the world go away, the only thing left is to disappear yourself? Anorexia – far from being about looking slim – is a severe form of punishment, of self-hatred and deep psychological distress. Children say with their bodies what they can't say with words.

Nobody knows why Olivia was unlucky enough to get sick. Numerous studies have shown that perfectionism is more prevalent in children suffering from anorexia nervosa and certain other eating disorders. And Olivia is a bright child. *Gifted*, her dad, Matthew, tells me. 'She's brilliant at the violin already.' But other children are perfectionist and don't get eating disorders. There is so much that we don't understand – but that doesn't help Matthew, who tells the nurses that he and Olivia's mum feel as if it is their fault somehow. The nurses try and reassure them, but Matthew is holding back tears. A big man, he's stooped over, as if avoiding a low ceiling. It's Olivia's mum, Alexandra, who looks most broken, though.

The nurses are gearing Olivia up to spend the day at home with her mum on her birthday, but it's clearly causing anxiety for them both. Alexandra fusses around her daughter, plaiting her dry, wispy hair, putting in colourful bobbles. 'Do you want purple? Or green? It's a lovely blue.' She holds up the colourful hair accessories one by one, as if they are fragile and full of meaning. The more choice she gives Olivia, the less Olivia can make a decision. It's a painful dance between them. Eventually Alexandra puts green bobbles in Olivia's hair and smiles broadly. 'There. Beautiful.' And I notice that her hands are shaking. Alexandra sits down on the edge of the bed and starts talking about family members, filling Olivia in on life outside the hospital. 'Your teachers send their love,' she says. 'They're looking forward to you going back to school very soon. I mean, I know you have school here every day with your activities, but I mean normal school.' The word 'normal' hangs sharply in the air and Alexandra opens her mouth slightly, as if she's hoping the word will travel back into it.

But Olivia snuggles up beside her and changes course. She has recognised the anxiety in her mum, and the tension and pain. 'Green is still my favourite colour,' she says, touching the bobbles in her hair.

I've subscribed to *Be My Parent* and *Children Who Wait* and have a collection: a stack of babies, children and sibling groups, all with smiling photos, short descriptions underneath, much like those at the adoption party. It is so odd, flicking through a catalogue of children, trying not to imagine the sadness they must have suffered. I look at the faces and want to take them all home. But I also want all children to have the chance to live with their birth parents, whenever possible. I worry that they simply haven't been given the help they need, the support we all deserve. I have heard stories about what these birth families have been through. I want to go back in time – take them home, too. But, I realise, adoption is sometimes the only hope of changing the course of one child's life. Breaking a cycle of tragedy.

We get almost daily emails from our social worker – a different one now, whose job is 'matching': that is, matching a child to the right family, and a family to the right child. She calls and messages: *Can you consider this child? This baby? Read this CPR [Child Permanence Report] form?* Often she attaches a photograph, or there is a photograph and information in the CPR, which also contains the basic background on what led the child into care, and what birth-family history they have and are able to share. I find it dizzying, reading about children who need families. I study the forms very carefully, reading between the lines, and try to imagine how my birth daughter will cope with a particular child's issues. And think about how I will cope supporting a child. I often ask for more information. And I dream about all these children, waiting for a for-ever family. Then one day I receive a phone call: 'I've sent you an email, in error – another CPR. Just delete it. It's a child, a boy, but he's all the way in Scotland. So just delete it.'

Something in her voice makes my ears prick up. The words don't match what lies underneath. Clever people, social workers. I open the email. And suddenly there he is. My son, aged two, looking at me with wide-open eyes. I know instantly that this child is my son. Nature–nurture doesn't matter. He's completely my son. I feel it in my bones, my gut, the back of my head and somewhere below my ribs. All the other children I have seen and wanted to help now evaporate. I am in love in a second. I am reminded so clearly of the day my daughter was born, curled up in a hedgehog ball, and of the enormity of love that I felt. How could I feel a love like that again? Yet here it is.

He likes to dance! He likes music! And being outside! He loves to throw balls! I want to lift him out of the photograph and wrap him inside my arms for always. I cry and cry. I long to hold him. Simply seeing my son's face reminds me that in the darkness of life there are flashes of the most beautiful golden light. I hope I am good enough. I think of my daughter. How will she cope with a sibling? One not born to me? But something gives me confidence that she'll do better than cope. It's as if she was born to be a sister. I imagine she will perform magic that I don't quite understand.

I print the photo of her brother-to-be and show it to her, and she takes it and stares at it for the longest of times, holding it tightly in her hand. I retrieve it gently and put it on the mantelpiece. But later it is missing. I ask my daughter where it is, and she denies all knowledge. I search and search, getting cross. I can't find it anywhere. Eventually I give up and reprint the photo; I am desperate to gaze at his face. The following morning I find the photo underneath my daughter's pillow. When she says it 'magicked there', I laugh, but then her face becomes serious and thoughtful and I wonder if she is going to voice a worry. But she frowns a fraction. 'I dreamed my brother last night,' she says. 'He told me that we have to get a dog. A guinea pig. Or a hamster. We have to. Or he doesn't want to live with us.'

Before leaving hospital to visit home, Olivia wafts around, tissue-paper-like, a husk of a child. I try and chat with her, suggest a game of Snap or a slow walk in the sunshine, but she's listless and preoccupied. Until Toby arrives, that is.

Toby is eleven and has pulled out his eyebrows and eyelashes and most of his hair, and is wearing a cloak over his T-shirt. He has come to the unit as an outpatient and lives at home with his sisters, his parents and a hamster called Batman. Today the nurses have agreed that Batman can accompany him for his treatment – art therapy, counselling, medication, further assessment, care plans.

Olivia and Toby fist-bump and move into a secret hand-shake that they have apparently developed over the course of their short friendship. She smiles and I notice her tiny yellow teeth, her reddened gums. But then I see the smile reach her eyes and something changes inside her. She glows. In the living-room area, Toby takes Batman out and puts him in a

Perspex ball. Olivia and Toby follow the hamster round as he crashes into everything: the chair legs, the wall, the table. The entire time they talk in a made-up language. 'Banana language,' Olivia tells me. 'You wouldn't understand.'

I sip a cup of tea and watch them – two children obviously delighted in each other – and smile to myself. And at lunchtime Olivia sits next to Toby and eats, without much drama. Another nurse tells me that mealtimes are fraught with emotion and panic and it's our job to keep things friendly and relaxed, and not focus too much on food, but rather on experience. But Olivia and Toby eat with their mouths open, talking nonsensical language, and laugh at Batman banging around underneath the table in his Perspex ball.

After lunch Olivia laughs and picks up Batman in his ball, squealing with delight as she frees him. 'There you go, Batman. That's better. We don't like being trapped, do we?'

Toby giggles hysterically. 'You and Batman are both prisoners,' he says.

And Olivia pauses, screws her face up slightly, then lifts Batman to eye level in the palm of her hand. 'We're the same,' she whispers.

People often ask me, as a writer, if writing from a child's perspective is easier. It's much harder. To access the voice of a child means climbing inside memory, forgetting in order to remember. Perhaps, in a similar way, to understand child and adolescent mental health properly you need to be a child.

Academics, researchers, clinicians, esteemed and experienced practitioners working in mental health are still a long way from understanding the treatments that might work best for children. But eleven-year-old Toby knows what helps Olivia most: banana language, a best friend and a hamster named Batman.

7

I Got You Babe

I wish I could say that giving my brother an LSD acid tab when he was fourteen years old and I was fifteen, for doing the washing up, is the most stupid thing I've ever done. But it probably isn't.

My dad and I are eating Chinese food and I'm now an adult. It's mid-June and there's a tree in full bloom next to us. We sit outside, so Dad can smoke. He blows giant clouds of smoke as though he's Gandalf in *Lord of the Rings*. We're having a heart-to-heart and we're both a bit drunk, which is when we talk most. I want to tell him about the stupid things I've done, and other important bigger stuff, but I find myself staring at the tree. It's hard to talk. The blossom and my dad's smoke remind me of X-rays of children that I care for: patchy soft clouds of disease. I can't separate myself from my nursing any longer. The two are fused. Eventually I do talk and the words come out in a rush. I tell him about the drugs, and how I could have harmed my beloved brother so much.

'I don't know why I did it, or what I was thinking. It seemed normal. I didn't even take anything myself. I have no idea why I thought it was okay.' I close my eyes. The things that seemed normal to my messed-up teenage brain.

'It was just a trip.' My dad shrugs. 'You were probably conceived on a Purple Om.' He laughs and I don't know if he's laughing because it's a joke, or because it happened. It would explain a lot. I know my dad has a pretty relaxed attitude to drugs. He used to grow weed in the airing cupboard for a while, and after my friend died by suicide when I was twenty-one, he gave me something to smoke that he called Rocky Death Black, and claimed it would knock me out for far longer than any prescription sedative. 'I think it's best for you not to be fully conscious until the funeral. Get back on track afterwards.' I sobbed into his jumper until it was soaked.

I'm in a perpetual state of confusion, grief and shock about my behaviour during my teenage years. My 'going off the rails as a teenager' is a subject that peppers every chat between my mum and me to this day. I spent the years between thirteen and sixteen putting myself in dangerous situations, hanging around with much older friends who were also low-level criminals. Before nursing, I lived a life of chaos. I was self-destructive, but it seemed completely normal. I used to think that nursing saved my life, with its rules and structure and kind people. But those older friends were not unkind. They treated me like a sister and were full of moral codes, with a list of ethics longer than the nurses' Code of Professional Conduct. Both my wayward youth and my nursing made me who I am today: not a devil, or an angel, but a complicated person made of light and dark – as we all are – doing my best to be better. I hope I am learning.

Harming myself during that time is one thing; potentially harming my brother, whom I adore and always have, is beyond my understanding, though. He is almost exactly a year younger than me and for a while we are even in the same class at school. We grow up to be inseparable. Almost every single memory I have of my early childhood contains my brother.

'Why would I do that?' I take another sip of wine.

My dad takes a puff and blows out more clouds. He leans back on the wooden chair. 'I wouldn't worry about it,' he says. 'And don't tell me anything else. Mistakes and regrets are between you and the moon.' He has a way with words, my dad. And he understands silence. But this silence feels dangerous.

I think about all the directions my life could have taken. Of friends who ended up in and out of prison. And how it could easily have been my dad. Or me.

I look at my dad, with the moon behind him.

'Michael is a twenty-three-weeker in bed six, bay two. His dad's in prison, and his mum is in a facility needing round-the-clock care following a traumatic brain injury. Michael's had a grade-four intraventricular haemorrhage overnight and has been unstable on dopamine, and his gases are impressive: we need to put him back on the oscillator this morning. We've been trying to organise for his dad, Danny, to get day-release to visit.' She pauses. 'He kicked the pregnant mum in the stomach, then threw her down the stairs. She landed on concrete.'

Like the other nurses and student nurses sitting in the staffroom for handover, I shake my head a fraction, but carry on scribbling down the vital information onto the handover sheet. The nurse in charge is an advanced neonatal nurse practitioner who has night-shift breath that I can smell from a fair distance: coffee, pear drops. Along with varicose veins, bad backs and, too often, PTSD symptoms, coffee-breath is an almost inevitable and unpleasant side-effect of the job.

She pauses a beat, then carries on. She's seen it all before – and some. 'Christie, can you look after him, please? If they agree to the visit, the dad will be accompanied by a prison officer, so we'll need to make some room around the bed space, and be conscious of the other parents.'

I nod, but my knees shake. The oscillator machine that delivers ventilation to the sickest of all babies is a scary thing, as is caring for a premature baby with a severe bleed in his brain, who needs drugs so strong they can be dangerous: dopamine and adrenaline infusions. Perfect mathematics and technical skills are crucial. But it is not those things that worry me.

Kicked in the stomach and thrown down the stairs.

What kind of monster does that? And how will I not let him see that I think he's a monster? I don't consider for a second that perhaps he is not a monster. Or that all our lives are shaped by our circumstances. Instead I feel the colour of my own blood: violent, angry red.

I pray to any god I can think of that they won't let the man out to see his son and that I can simply concentrate on caring for Michael, which will be work enough. Other units and wards seem to alternate between calm and busy, but not Special Care Baby Units (SCBUs) or Neonatal Intensive Care Units (NICUs). NICU is busy all year round and in July, without fail, it is hot – hotter than you could imagine. NICU means throwing open the doors and not stopping; it means thinking and doing and running for twelve and half hours straight. I like being so busy that you look up at the clock at 8 a.m. and suddenly it's late afternoon and you have no idea how it happened. The babies' hearts beat frantically, and the day mirrors that. And perhaps it is the pull of nature that makes the wildness and unpredictability of these babies – these almost humans – seem like a storm blown in from nowhere, reminding the nurses they are not in charge after all. One minute the numbers on the machines tell the nurses that everything is fine, stable, and the next minute there's a bleed in the brain, a necrotic section of bowel, a life-threatening infection. In NICU, premature babies are nurtured until they are ready for the world and anything can go wrong until then: intussusception, meningitis, sepsis, seizures, pneumonia, necrotising enterocolitis. I have looked after babies with bits born outside them: their guts, kidneys, brain. And babies who have bits the wrong way around inside them: hearts, kidneys, intestines.

Then there are the parents. Anyone can have a premature baby at any time, and we won't always know why. But there are high-risk groups more prone to prematurity, and the ward is full of vulnerable women: young, poor, drug-addicted, refugees, women who've miscarried again and again and again and again. A fourteen-year-old girl comes in with suspected appendicitis and gives birth in the hospital toilet. A woman suffering from depression has scars all down her arms, and a mental health nurse is brought in to care for her alongside the nurses caring for her baby. Another woman had a stillbirth last year, and lost twins the year before. Through the armhole of the incubator she holds her daughter's impossibly small hand in her fingertips as she stares at the monitor, her face empty.

The newcomers are hyper-alert, hooked up to catheters or in wheelchairs pushed straight from Caesarean sections or post-natal wards, but most mothers are here for the long haul, spending four months-plus on the same ward, in the same heat, the same noise. They get to know the nurses so well they can tell them apart by the sound of their footsteps along the corridor, and they either breathe a sigh of relief or start to panic – the life of their baby in the hands of someone they do not trust as much as others. And the nurses know the mothers well enough to be relieved or totally dreading a shift, depending on who they are looking after. The baby is never the issue.

Things are not as nature intended here: babies are spoken about in terms of corrected or adjusted ages that take into account the date they were meant to arrive, so a ten-week-old baby eight weeks early is 'two weeks corrected'. The nurses keep these babies alive until the date they were due to be born, with technology, drugs and care, and in doing so try and 'correct' nature. But they do a lot more than that, too. Many of the babies here are four months away from being their 'corrected' ages. Their mothers would perhaps not even have looked pregnant yet. The births that some of the mothers describe are the most traumatic of all. They tell me of the sweaty panic of waking in the night to a wet patch on the sheets and wondering if it's blood or amniotic fluid, or both. The babies arrive to bright lights and medical procedures, and everyone holding their breath. They go from a warm, floating and calm environment, to doctors and nurses inserting endotracheal tubes into tiny mouths and noses; or umbilical venous lines, attaching monitoring until so little of the baby is visible that they begin to appear robotic, not human at all.

The nurses place miniature knitted hats on the babies' fragile heads and stick their hospital identification bands around their minuscule limbs, or on the outside of the incubators. And then they all wait for the time when the babies are not meant to be here to pass – a dance in between life and birth and death. In some countries the nurses carry the premature babies around in what are called kangaroo pouches. It makes sense to me as an idea for babies who come too early. Of course our incubators act as a sort of womb, but the truth is that I would love to have a baby in a pouch as I work. I am obsessed with babies. I love their smell, their small movements, their yawns and stretches. I also love their fast-running hearts, their ability to bounce back, their will to survive, their minuscule tubes, umbilical catheters, delicate tissue-paper skin, both fragile and powerful at once.

I walk through the ward, past the fridges and thank-you cards and infection-control notices; the poster that encourages staff well-being; and the sign-up sheet for yoga and meditation, which makes me smile even though I'm anxious. There is something written on it that has been crossed out, but you can still see the words underneath: *I didn't have time to pee for twelve hours yesterday. Namaste.*

Michael is in the main bay area, where the lights are bright and the babies are sick and the nurses are rushing around, biros poked through their hurried ponytails, calculations worked out on the backs of their dry, hard-working nurses' hands. He is hooked up to every machine imaginable – all big, chugging, complex technology with him in the middle: a little dot like a full stop in the centre of a chemistry textbook. He has all the trappings of prematurity: lungs that do not yet produce enough surfactant, a gut that does not yet absorb food properly, poor reflexes, no suck reflex, a lack of temperature control. He has suffered the worst kind of bleed to his brain. He also has retinopathy of prematurity, the eye condition that caused Stevie Wonder's blindness. But these conditions don't paint the picture of him. When I first meet Michael, I notice the downy hair that I recognise from caring for teenagers suffering from anorexia, and from Olivia. His skin is almost entirely see-through, and his entire foot is the size of my thumbnail. He has a permanent frown, which makes him look like a grumpy old man, and he smells of yoghurt.

'He's the size of half a bag of sugar, but he is oh-so-mighty and has dodged death so many times that we call him "the mouse with nine lives".' One of the nurses, Grainne, is giving a handover – another handover – at the bedside. She has written *Mighty Mouse* on his whiteboard. 'We shouldn't have favourites,' she says, as if she's talking about her own children, 'but he's mine.'

She tells me about his history in his short three days of life, which is more than most of us will ever go through: Michael has had the worst start imaginable. Born addicted to crack cocaine and heroin, even in his tiny state he shows signs of foetal alcohol syndrome: characteristic facial features and a small head circumference known as microcephaly. Like all the babies on NICU, his story started before he did. Some children are born with odds stacked so high against them it's impossible to comprehend any meaningful recovery, and yet nursing has taught me that recovery is always a possibility; there is always hope.

Michael's 'Mighty Mouse' nickname hints that he might have the will to survive, to fulfil Grainne's hope that he'll be one of the lucky few. 'I've been singing to him all night – I think my voice made him frown.' She laughs. But it's these things that nurses do, which supposedly make no sense, that make the most sense to me. Along with delivering expert and evidence-based care, supporting his multi-organ failure and resuscitating him, she prescribes him songs and nursery rhymes. I wonder if he can hear her. I hope so.

I wash my hands and carefully untangle Michael from all the tubes and wires to pick him up as gently as possible. It's like holding air. I want to leave him alone as much as possible for the day, to rest and grow, but his skin is so thin he's at risk of marks and pressure sores. He is shaking. He has been having seizures, which we treat with Lorazepam delivered via a small archaic machine that is set by fiddling with a dial using a pair of scissors. The amount of times I have cut my hand trying to set up the Lorazepam machine is ridiculous (there are better alternatives nowadays).

It turns out that Michael's shaking is not a seizure; it is withdrawal. Drug-addicted babies are a regular feature of NICUs. Every single thing that most pregnant women do as a matter of course – prenatal vitamins, not smoking, not drinking, not taking drugs, sufficient rest, reducing stress – is almost impossible if you are a mum dealing with substance misuse and mental-health conditions, or both. But of all the things that have affected Michael during his mum's pregnancy, I would imagine stress is the worst. While other babies hear soothing voices, he must have been on high alert, being kicked and shouted at before he was even born, absorbing the stress that his mother endured. Domestic violence often happens for the first time during pregnancy, or escalates if it was already happening. The unborn baby is at risk of stress, anxiety, prematurity, infection and death. Midwives and nurses continually ask about domestic violence and abuse throughout a woman's pregnancy, but of course some women never see a midwife or have contact with a nurse.

Years later I'm visiting a prison, and thinking back to Michael's dad, Danny. The prison nurses tell me that nobody is born bad, and a person can't be judged on a single event, no matter how horrible the crime they've committed. I learn about the issues the nurses deal with here, the complex decisions that involve them. These nurses are unflappable and calm in every possible crisis.

'It's the most autonomous area of nursing I can think of.' Gill, the prison nurse, has a soft voice. He's wearing a uniform and a belt, attached to which is a giant pair of keys. But he radiates warmth and smiles continuously, which is not how I imagined a prison nurse to be. I'd pictured someone serious, formal. But Gill is friendly, relaxed and chatty. 'We're nurse-led. The career progression is limitless, and we deal with all aspects of health that you can imagine, from mental-health crises to end-of-life care, to substance misuse. And some of these people's lives … It's hard to imagine they would end up anywhere else.' His face changes for a second, becomes thoughtful, and there is a flicker of anguish. 'These poor men.' And there is sympathy and empathy etched across his skin.

I see how much Gill cares about the inmates, and about inequality. I learn from him that 27 per cent of prisoners have been looked after in the care system. Black men are 26 per cent more likely than white men to be remanded in custody. As the mother of a black son who was previously 'looked after' (in care), I find these statistics truly shocking and horrifying. As a human being, I find them truly shocking and horrifying. As a nurse? Sadly, I am not remotely surprised. Even in nursing, the inequalities are vast. And nurses daily see the division and inequality in our society, the people hidden from view. The people cared for, regardless of all else, by Gill and nurses like him. I meet so many inspirational nurses. And I find them in unusual places.

Nurses work with every single kind of person. Within our society there is a giant safety net made up of nurses, social workers and police and prison officers. They catch the most vulnerable people among us. Beneath that, there are the nurses working on the ground with those who have fallen through even that last net. Nurses working in justice and forensic healthcare, for example, work in police custody suites and prisons, and secure units and immigration detention centres, and with those who have suffered sexual violence, and yet also with those who have been violent. I wonder what draws nurses to this specialised area of work? How do they remain non-judgemental?

The idea of forensic nursing leaves me cold. I don't want to take a penile swab from a potential rapist or make other similar interventions. But one of the brightest and most talented nurses I meet explains a draw to forensic nursing that I hadn't previously considered. Jess, a member of the Queen's Nursing Institute Scotland (QNIS), is a shining light. She is the kind of nurse – and person – I want to be. The QNIS and its partner organisation based in London, the Queen's Nursing Institute (QNI), are charities with the vision that all people deserve the best possible nursing care, by the right nurse, with the right skills, in homes and communities, whenever and wherever necessary. The QNI works with community nurses and is probably the oldest professional nursing organisation in the UK, maybe even the world. Queen's Nurses from the QNI and QNIS work in all manner of settings: as district nurses, homeless health nurses, in primary care, health visiting, school nursing, learning disability and mental-health settings, and form a national network of nurse leaders, publishing research and influencing policy-makers.

I am lucky enough to have met many impressive Queen's Nurses, but Jess is next level. She exudes leadership. Just being around her reassures me. It must reassure her patients and colleagues, too. 'Our job is to make sure people are in the best health possible, safe, well fed, physically and mentally looked after and cared for, in order that they are fit to face the Court so the accused and the complainant can get truth and justice.' I had never considered that forensic nursing in police custody or prison would have as much influence over the trial as the criminal defence barrister, but of course, as ever, there is a quiet power in nursing. 'It helps that we think about human rights and entire lives, rather than one big terrible moment. No person is all good or all bad.'

I spend some time with nurses in a police custody suite. The rooms are yellow and blue with heavy multi-bolted metal doors, and whiteboards above them displaying the name of the person inside, separated into men's and women's corridors. I go inside a cell. The toilet is shaped like a cone, 'in case of removal of DNA evidence with water, or potential self-harm', and there is a smell that is much like certain wards in hospitals: fetid humanity covered in bleach. In the small kitchen I see the food for people waiting in cells: cardboard trays of dried chicken or some Pot Noodles. Most people opt for the latter, I'm told, but a mix of both the chicken and noodles is apparently good at reversing diabetic hypoglycaemic low blood-sugar attacks. I wonder what Omar, in cell one, thinks of the Pot Noodles, and whether they are halal. Or if they're just generally bad for you.

Like all other areas of nursing, both in and out of hospital, safe staffing is a difficult aspect of Jess's job: not enough nurses, police officers or social workers to deal with the work. 'Many of the people who end up in places like this are disenfranchised and marginalised, and may not go near a GP,' she says. 'We try to bring the help they need to them. Some of these people lead desperate lives.' Jess doesn't moan, but quietly goes about her day and makes improvements as she goes. Laughing whenever she can and, when she can't, holding it behind her eyes. She has that nurse's look that I recognise: stoic, slightly sarcastic and, most of all, resilient.

All her nurses are trained prescribers, able to give opiate replacement therapy and other medicines to help prevent people addicted to drugs going into withdrawal. It's a no-brainer, but it's made a massive difference. I wonder why this is not standard for all police custody and prison nurses in the UK. Jess tells me about the huge increase in violence that she has seen in her daily work, particularly rape cases. Some of her work involves caring for rape complainants and alleged assailants. I don't know how she does it. But I'm glad she does. We should all be glad of nurses like Jess, who believe in justice and humanity and the bigger picture. The pursuit of truth.

*

'These men can have their entire lives judged on a single snap-shot.' Gill is walking me through the long, thin corridors, which might as well be hospital corridors. He picks up on me looking at the cleaner who is polishing the floor. 'Same smell as hospital, right? All the same product and equipment, from the same suppliers.' The smell is identical: a cheap, faintly chlorinated bleach that has dried with the windows closed. The walls are painted the same dull yellow, too: I wonder if the paint is also produced by the same supplier. Eventually, after many winding corridors, we arrive at the medical centre, which should really be called the nursing centre. 'We offer mental-health and phys-ical-health services, all the clinics you can imagine, from group therapy to a blood-borne disease service. It's autonomous and holistic, and one of the safest places to nurse.'

I discover that the men here are split into different categories, and are never allowed to cross paths with other categories in case they attack one another. 'The paedophiles are the easiest to manage. We're allowing them to have a bird cage, but we couldn't do that with any of the other pris-oners.' I learn that the prisoners with paedophilic personality disorders are often from a certain demographic: white, middle-class, middle-aged. 'The kind of men you might find in suburban garden centres,' a healthcare assistant tells me.

I watch Gill in his office. He's a band-six nurse, which is one rung up from newly qualified, yet he commands the respect of all the nurses in the team. His office looks like any other nurse's – a rota on the wall, a list of staff clinics and the opening times of the GP practice – and you would not know it is inside a prison.

He tells me it's not the prison population that causes the stress in prison. It's nearly always conflicts or communication difficulties between the nurses and the prison officers. Their relationships are improving, but they have such different perspectives.

I learn much from Gill and his team. I learn how people develop jail habits: becoming addicted to drugs while in prison – the drugs arriving by drone, or thrown over the wall inside dead rats, or soaked into clothing, which is then subsequently washed and the water collected and ingested somehow. I learn how many people in prison have an undiagnosed or untreated personality disorder. How vulnerable prisoners are. How many of the prisoners have addiction issues and underlying mental illnesses, and horrific childhood experiences. People are not born bad. Each and every one of us makes mistakes. Morality is even more complicated in prison. Nurses must care for everyone, regardless of their past, even those displaying the most extreme sides of human behaviour. Still, it's hard not to judge.

'Some of our friends here have convictions for violent crimes, rapes, murders. We leave all that at the door. If we judge them, we won't have time to love them.'

I am meeting someone described to me by many nurses as 'the kindest nurse in Britain'. Rachel, a parish nurse working with homeless people, has a direct gaze, as if looking inside me, right into my bones. It's at once unnerving and strangely comforting. She looks at everyone she speaks to like that, I notice. We are in a church and there is home-made lentil soup, and each person gets a roll, a yoghurt and tea or coffee. 'Macaroni cheese is the best,' a woman tells me. She is, like all the visitors here, homeless and a drug addict (or substance abuser, or self-medicating or, even better, a person, Rachel corrects me). When I ask about the toilets, I'm told there are none, because the risk of people overdosing in them is so high.

'Brilliant macaroni,' the woman continues. Her eyes are not focusing, but she seems coherent in her speech. She is obsessed with Hello Kitty and has the most perfectly groomed eyebrows I've ever seen. She shows me the map that Rachel designed to make it easier for homeless people to find and access services in the city. 'I mean, it seems obvious – an actual map and directions – but no one else had done it.'

So much of nursing, I think to myself, seems obvious, and yet seeing that need in the first place is difficult and takes experience, training and something extra. She's as high as a kite, this woman, and doesn't eat any of her soup, but it's clear how much she respects these nurses. She scratches and twitches and leans against a skinny man who has a tattoo on his face. She can't look directly at anyone, I notice. Her eyes dart and dance around the room as if she's terrified they'll land in one place. I thought at first it was because she was intoxicated, but it's more than that. When I make a flicker of eye contact with her, it's enough to see her absolute pain.

'We don't call them service users. God, I hate that term.' Barbara is also a parish nurse. She's been here 'donkey's years' and, already way past retirement, will probably never leave. 'These are our friends. Our family. We're no better than they are. Any one of us who'd had their lives would be in their position. We've known some of them twenty years. And at least one member of our family dies every single week. We go to a lot of funerals.'

So many nurses go to a lot of funerals. But to know a person for twenty years and consider them family, and lose someone every week, takes a courage that I can't imagine. The courage of nurses.

A woman with knowing eyes, Ruth, hands me a laughing baby while she gets some baby food out of a pushchair.

'She's gorgeous,' I say. And she is. Fat, happy and smiling, and charming every single person who tickles her under the chin.

Ruth kisses the baby, who squeals in delight. She opens a jar of baby food and feeds her daughter tenderly, spoon by spoon, making noises as it goes towards her delighted face.

The baby looks at her mum exactly as a baby should look at a mum – with total unconditional love. I ask Ruth about the parish nurses.

'I was in prison and Barbara came to see me every week on her day off. She didn't miss a visit. Helped me to stay clean and be a good mum.'

I look over at Barbara. She has pink hair and wears a cross around her neck. In a few years' time I'll attend an awards ceremony and she will get a lifetime-achievement award from QNIS, and even then Barbara won't like any fuss. I'll meet her husband, who says he's long-suffering as she simply won't retire, but who looks at her with such love and pride that I can't stop staring.

I turn back to Ruth. 'How was prison?' I ask.

'I loved it. They looked after me. Best place I've ever lived.'

I close my mouth, realising it has fallen open. What must life have been like for this woman, to say that prison is the best place she's ever lived? Rachel tells me that 25–50 per cent of homeless people were once in care. These people bounce around a system that fails them from the moment they are born, finally ending up in a place like this, where there is no longer any safeguarding. They are at rock-bottom, and the nurses – and each other – are sometimes all they have.

I think of my son. I think of his birth mother.

Barbara walks past and pinches the baby's cheek. There is so much love in this room that the air feels sticky with it.

After lunch we do karaoke. We sing cringe-worthy ballads and pop songs and everyone joins in, including the staff, including me. There's a large television screen showing the words, but most of the clients look at each other, smiling, happy and present in the moment. It's the most eye contact I've seen from any of them. Rachel stands at the front with a client and they perform a duet of 'I Got You Babe', and they are simply two women having the best time, teasing each other about their dance moves. There is grace in this room as well as laughter – something divine. Perhaps this is exactly what churches should be. What they are for. A sign on the wall says: *Love Thy Neighbour*. There are no conditions underneath it. It doesn't say: *Love Thy Neighbour (if they look like you and sound like you, and especially if they are not mad, bad, or dangerous)*. I'm singing as hard as I can, in my terrible voice, and Ruth whoops over at me and, grinning, sticks her thumb in the air. Her baby is balanced on her hip and is the happiest that a baby has ever been.

I watch them all. But I am mesmerised by Rachel. I watch her total delight in making others happy. Helping them feel whole, like someone with value and hope and joy. She loves them. And they love her. She is truly the kindest nurse in the UK.

The people in this room, which is full of rough sleepers and addicts and criminals, dance and sing and are transported to a safe, happy place, and for a short time they are not rough sleepers and addicts and criminals, or even patients or service users. Rachel is right. They are just people. Like me, like you. And even like Michael's dad, Danny.

Danny is handcuffed to a prison officer and is next to Michael's incubator when I return from breakfast at 4 p.m., my first break of the day. The prison officer and Danny have a similar look: hard-looking men with shit tattoos. I expect to hate Danny. Being non-judgemental towards abusers is so difficult, and I've learned to hate and judge while keeping a poker face. I smile at him and explain the tubes and wires and the situation. 'Michael's had a very rough few days.' I tell Danny about the cardiac arrests, the bleed in his brain, the fight in him.

Danny laughs at the *Mighty Mouse* written on the side of Michael's chart, but he rubs it off and writes *Mike Tyson* instead. 'Little fighter, like me,' he says.

And I smile at this monster.

I find a chair for Danny and for the prison guard, Sam, who despite his hard-edged face is as soft-voiced and calm as a nurse. They both sit and marvel over Michael, as I feed him donated milk through a nasogastric tube. I am particularly careful with testing this before putting any milk in, using blue litmus paper to check the acid confirming that the tube is in his stomach – rather than (as with another baby on the ward recently) going accidentally up into the skull and wrapping around his brain. Nowadays, thankfully, nasogastric tubes are usually X-rayed to check they are in the right position.

'I was born early too.' Danny is stroking Michael's head in the softest way possible. 'A small bag of sugar.' He looks up at me. 'Six foot two now.'

'It's a strange phenomenon that ex-premmies often end up so tall,' I say. We both look at Michael. He is extremely unlikely to survive. There is a time for bad news and a time for hope, and this may be the only time that father and son spend together. Michael's mum is deteriorating, hence Danny being allowed to visit them both today. Whatever happens, he'll be in prison for a long time. If Michael survives, he will end up in the care system; and if his mum survives, she will be in a care setting too, requiring years of rehab.

Michael is stable on the oscillator and his numbers look good. He is not yet well enough to come out of the incubator, but I encourage Danny to touch him anyway, to talk to him and sing to him.

He cracks up laughing at the suggestion of singing, but does put his hand gently underneath Michael's miniature body and lifts him slightly as I pull the corner of his special sheet to make sure there are no creases. There is a moment, between the two of them. Michael is curled into the palm of his dad's hand. The light changes. Danny's eyes change. It's as though they were both born for this one moment. And it's maybe these moments that connect us all. These extreme moments of love that shock us out of who we are and remind us of who we could be.

I quietly slip round to the other side of the bed space and take a photo with one of the instant cameras that are always kept on NICU, for when a photo urgently needs to be taken. Usually when a baby is close to dying. I take two photos. One of Danny's face, and then a close-up of Michael, curled up in Danny's hand.

It's a short visit and when it's time to go, I give Danny the photos. He looks at the photo of Michael in his hand and he is crying. 'I'll treasure this, Nurse.'

And I see that he will. And that this photo has instantly become the most important thing he owns. It does not allow me to feel any pity for him, but he is no longer a monster to me. Just a weak man, a bit pathetic. A man with no power at all.

'Wait,' I tell him. I disappear and come back with the camera. 'Can you wash your hands and hold him carefully again.'

Danny does so and again sits next to Michael. He picks him up and I get the photo – almost exactly the same as the first one. Michael's heart rate, which was much too high, falls at the touch of Danny's hand. His father leans towards him and sings, off-key, a few lines of 'Danny Boy'.

I wonder if a man ever sang that song to Danny. If that's how he got his name. And what kind of man he was.

*

Like teachers, nurses can't influence who a person becomes as much as their parents can. We cannot change someone's fate, the cards they are dealt. Even so, after Danny leaves, I wipe the words *Mike Tyson* from Michael's whiteboard. I stick the extra photo to the top of his incubator and write at the top: *Important. Please keep*, along with the date and Danny's name. I write on the whiteboard:

Michael, son of Danny and Hannah.

8

Basketball Player

The day we're due to meet my son's birth parents, I wake at sunrise. I focus on a spider's web outside my bedroom window: perfectly ordered lines against the brightening sky.

In an adoption information evening we were given a ball of wool and told to sit in different places around the room. I held the end of the wool. 'Imagine you are the child who is being adopted,' the social worker told me. Then she unwound the wool and asked someone else to hold it, 'Imagine you are the social worker'; and another, 'You are the foster carer' and 'You are the birth grandparent', and so on and so on until there were so many lines of wool it became a spider's web. A complex and beautiful structure of all the people who love someone and are involved in their life. Then she came back to me, holding all these connections, and she cut through everything with a giant pair of scissors. She handed a piece of wool to me, a single strand, and gave one end of it to a woman behind me. A stranger I could not see. 'Every single person you have ever known and loved is gone. Every one of them. Not just birth parents, but also birth aunty, grandparents, teacher, nursery nurse, neighbour, social worker, foster carer, foster sibling. Everyone. And now you have a new connection. Brand-new – with a stranger – and everyone else is gone.'

I spend almost two hours deciding what to wear. Ridiculous. But I want nothing to make it worse than it has to be. I know I can't make it better, so not making it worse is my ultimate aim. My 'matching' social worker keeps telling me, 'This will be very hard. Maybe the hardest thing you ever do.' She repeats it like a mantra, as if her responsibility is to make me truly understand in advance the emotions I might feel, which is of course impossible. And my clothing won't make a jot of difference. I think about how this woman must be feeling. Imagine losing a child. Having a child taken into care. It is too much to bear.

We're given a choice about meeting my son's birth parents. They want to meet us, to see where their son is going to live – who the powers-that-be have decided should raise their flesh and blood, until he is eighteen years old. At first, I refuse. No, I'm not strong enough. Plus, I think of the histories of children taken into care. I understand that when social workers and courts decide birth families are unable to keep their children safe, no matter how hard they've tried, it is always in the best interest of the child. Some families, even with vast support, are unable to parent a child in a way that any child deserves. I know all this. Yet I can also imagine the stories of birth families' own lives, and of their parents before them. My son's story began before I knew him, and he will be the one to explore it and choose if, and when, to share those details. But now I'm looking for certainty that I'm doing the right thing. Yet there is never any certainty in life. So while I'm unsure that I'll be able to deal with it, in the end I think of my son, and what will be best for him. Nothing, I realise, could ever make it 'best' – simply not worse. And meeting his birth parents will make it 'not worse'.

I have not yet met my son. Prospective adoptive parents don't get to meet their children until the process of moving in starts. Which is right: it is only when it will be for ever that a child should be introduced to a for-ever family. But I have more photos. A photograph of him eating cake – cake on his head and his cheeks and his hands. Another of him on a beach, with a bucket and spade beside him. Another of him with a cat on his lap. He has a cat that he loves, named Snowy. Both he and the cat are looking uncomfortable. He looks completely terrified in every single photo, something I don't notice until much later. 'Poor little man looks so afraid. Maybe he hates having his picture taken,' my mum says. Instead I focus on his dimples, the folds on his arms, his curly hair. I look at the photos so often they begin to rip at the edges, and I have to take more photos of the existing ones in case they get ruined. I want to keep the memories for him. The 'before'. His story.

I want to give him as many memories as possible. And for that I need details. Details that reports cannot give me. Gifts for my son. These are the only gifts that will truly matter to him as he grows, I already know that. I want to study his birth mother and his birth father even if only for a few minutes; and remember, remember, remember. But I am thinking most about his birth mum. A mother, like I am. As a nurse, I'm so used to walking in other people's shoes that I can't bear the thought of being in a room with her. I don't want to imagine her pain, wider than the sky.

But I want to know what she smells like, how she moves, the tone of her voice. Those things that make us. Of course I am worried I will feel anger as well as sadness. I may not yet have met my son, but I love him like the world has never seen love. Perhaps even stronger than that are my feelings of protectiveness towards him. He is only a toddler and yet his life has been disrupted, and no child should be scared of a cat on his lap. His eyes are wide open. He is on high alert, my son.

We meet at an office building, in a large, hot meeting room. My partner and I are with our social worker, and the birth parents will attend with theirs. I lean on my partner as we go into the room. There is a third social worker there, although I'm not sure why. As we walk over to the large table and chairs in the middle of the room, I glance at the window. Someone has drawn with a finger on one of the dirty windows:

a heart. I wonder who has drawn it: a child who has been in the room, or a birth family member; an adoptive mother like me, or a social worker like my mum. So many hearts spilling out in one place that anything is possible.

We are the first to arrive. We sit and make small talk with our social worker, but she keeps giving me really intense looks – to check that I am up to it, I imagine. I try so hard not to cry that my eyes feel dry and itchy.

She tells me again how today will work. Social workers like to explain everything in advance. I know they're trying to manage expectations, but I suspect it's more about attempting to take control of a situation where nobody has any control. There will be no handing over of a baby here, like in films or on TV. Adoption is nothing like that. Children in the UK are very rarely 'given up' by their birth parents. Children are taken into care. And they are not taken away lightly. 'There is no happy ending in adoption,' an adopted friend tells me. 'Just a different ending.'

My partner and I sit across from the birth parents and we both of us fake a smile and say hello. My partner is fidgeting, and I realise this is as hard for him as it is for me.

'Do you have any questions,' my social worker asks them. 'Anything at all?'

And they ask questions I had not expected.

Will you take him to church?

Will you teach him to cook?

The room feels hotter and hotter, and sweat drips down between my shoulder blades. The sun beats through the windows, and I can see a strip of blue sky outside.

It is a strange interview, on which so much depends. And I feel as if I'm failing in every sense. But then the time is up, and they stand to leave. My son's birth mother laughs out of nowhere. Snort-laughs. Then apologises. 'I laugh when I'm nervous,' she says. 'I don't know why.'

So we have one thing in common. I laugh too, and for a few seconds we are simply two women laughing. My partner look at us as if we have lost our minds.

Then we stop laughing.

Will you tell him about us?

'I promise,' I say, though the words sound so hollow.

Words are never enough. I feel a shot of pain in my stomach so powerful I almost double over. I have never felt anything like it in my life before. Everything blurs. My social worker sees it and moves next to me. My partner presses his leg against mine.

The social worker turns to the birth parents. 'Right, well, thank you so much for allowing this visit. It will really help your son, and I hope it's been helpful to you, too.'

Your son. *Your son. Your son.*

I focus on the window, and the outside behind her. Sometimes the sky is too blue.

I hold my breath as they walk out and, as the door shuts behind her, I fall to the ground and sob in waves that are beyond sadness.

'Adoption is joy that begins in tragedy,' my social worker reminds me.

And my partner holds me as I cry and cry, for this woman and this man who have no choice in this. I cry for my son who won't get to grow up with his birth parents. Perhaps I'm crying, too, for all the families of children I've cared for, who have lost a child. I watch the door after they have gone, and everything feels so wrong. I have never been less sure of anything, other than the pain these families feel: white-hot, searing pain. I always thought that childbirth must be the worst physical pain. I was wrong.

Jason is fifteen and has been stabbed repeatedly with a bread knife. He is known to be in a gang, and already has a violent past and boasts to nurses that he'll kill whoever did this. There are police officers at the end of the ward to prevent Jason leaving, and to stop gang members storming in (this happened once but, luckily, they were apprehended by security before getting to the children's ward) and committing some sort of revenge. We've also found a large serrated knife in his rucksack and some knuckledusters.

When I meet him, Jason is swearing and shouting. I try to find empathy for Jason somewhere inside me, but all I can see is an angry young man who carries weapons. And Jason appears stable, not seriously ill. His eyes are wide open, his voice is clear and sharp. His posture is normal, nor can I see much wrong with him physically. The numbers on the monitor are all within normal ranges for his age: blood pressure, oxygen levels, respiratory rate, heart rate. I can see the normal QRS pattern-waves on the monitor, suggesting that the electrics of his heart are fully functioning. Reading ECGs (electrocardiograms) is much like reading music. I take a few moments and watch the pattern that the electricity makes as it travels through his body, mesmerised as ever.

'I'm starving,' Jason shouts. 'I haven't eaten anything. I was on my way to get McDonald's when they came. I'm going to fuck them up.' His eyes are full of anger, but they show no signs of sickness: they are not distant, confused, glazed or sunken; there are no burst blood vessels. He's wearing jeans and his T-shirt has been cut off and is rolled up next to him. He clutches it now and then as if it's a soft toy. He has a rucksack – now empty of weapons – with his trainers inside it, and the police have his phone. There's a packet of chocolate Hobnobs in there too.

'You've got some biscuits in your bag,' I say, 'but you're nil by mouth until they've done all the X-rays and the scan. Later on you can eat them.'

He looks at me as if he wants to kill me. I have to hold in my mind that he's a child, and afraid. But I feel frightened.

Last month a junior nurse got punched in the face by an angry parent, leaving her with a broken eye socket. She did not press charges. 'They're losing a child,' she said. 'I'd want to punch someone if I'd had that sort of news.'

I'm already wondering if we can get Jason out of children's intensive care and to the children's ward, which accepts children from birth to eighteen years. If he kicks off here, there are critically ill children, and important pieces of kit everywhere. The child in the next bed space is on haemofiltration – a machine that acts as his kidneys, filtering all the blood of toxins, before replacing it in his body. Another child has an even more complicated machine: a MARS machine that acts as his liver. He is waiting for a liver transplant, and I don't know this yet, but he will teach me that children with liver disease bleed more than you could ever, ever imagine.

I'm qualified, and have been for many years, but I'm on a placement to learn different intensive-care skills at a trauma centre. This hospital specialises in trauma and transplants. There's a teenager with a bolt fixed through her skull across the ward; she had a head injury following a road-traffic accident that left her so hurt she arrived last week with brain coming through a skull fracture, like toothpaste being squeezed out through a tube. These are terrible things, but somehow over the years I am getting used to seeing the worst kinds of diseases and injuries. And in urban A&Es all staff are getting used to seeing children with stab injuries. These injuries increase in August – during the holidays children without the safety of school are far more vulnerable, with dangerous home situations, and knife crime amongst teens always increases then. Our understanding of this changes, though, with COVID-19. The Air Ambulance Team, which specialises in trauma and particularly in stabbings, is suddenly very quiet. No stabbings. Some of them are redeployed and work with critical-care patients and their families. Everyone is trying to make sense of gang behaviour – of everything we thought we knew.

August is also when A&E fills up with accidents, as opposed to diseases. Drunken picnics in the sun that lead to serious burn injuries; babies dehydrated from being left in cars; near-drownings in ponds and pools; people falling off bikes, or off buildings; people taking enough drugs at summer parties to kill a horse; broken bones and head injuries – including, once, a man almost beaten to death by his wife with a lawnmower.

I scan Jason's bed area. Everything matters. Every detail, every piece of equipment or drug in intensive care has the potential to harm – even kill – a patient. Intensive care provides life-support machines for children and adults in multi-organ failure, until their organs begin working again. But these machines can, and do, go wrong. I watch everything around Jason, checking and rechecking that the suction tubing is attached, that the bag valve mask has the correct-sized mask attached, that there are drugs drawn up and ready to go, should he need them, and that the dose is correct. Even knocking into the machine is a safety issue.

It's also a stupidly busy day, and we have no beds. 'No beds' doesn't necessarily mean literally no beds, but rather no nurses to look after a patient in those beds. Intensive-care nurses are safety-critical members of the workforce, and the specialist training takes many years. ICUs are far more than collections of equipment and ventilators; they cannot run without these specialist nurses. We are always short of intensive-care beds and nurses. There are vast inequalities in the funding of intensive care, and staff, across the world. In Germany there are 29.2 ICU beds per 100,000 members of the population; in the UK there are 6.6.

Today we've had to close beds to admissions in London, meaning that critically ill children will have to travel as far as Bristol, Liverpool or Southampton to get the specialist care they need. This journey puts their lives further at risk, and although there are no figures, it is fairly well understood that a long transfer of a seriously ill child increases their risk of death. No one should ever die in the back of an ambulance. As soon as we possibly can, we transfer children and young adults out of ICU and onto the wards, in order to free up beds. We try to have an intensive-care (or at least high-dependency) bed available for in-hospital children who deteriorate. Sometimes there's a patient having spinal surgery or complicated ENT (ear, nose and throat) surgery who will initially need a bed, post-op. And there are always those children who come in unexpectedly via A&E. Much of the work is thinking ten steps ahead, asking 'what if?' and prioritising. I work with a nurse from Ethiopia who tells me it's the opposite situation there. 'Here we take take the sickest. But they only have one bed in my local hospital – or at least the equipment – to manage one child needing intensive care, so they always prioritise the most well. The child likeliest to get better.'

To be on children's intensive care is brutal, but I'm constantly reminded of how lucky we are, and how privileged and narrow a speciality it is. It simply doesn't exist in other parts of the world. There are so many inequalities in our world. I'm also aware of the children's lives at home – the aftermath. How long recovery takes after time in ICU. Nobody walks out of intensive care. A spell on life-support leaves all kinds of long-term problems, ranging from PTSD and psychological disturbances, to hearing loss and serious and lifelong physical complications. I've cared for children in the community who are technology-dependent, completely reliant on life-support machines, or tracheostomies, or CPAP (continuous positive airway pressure) and other forms of ventilation, for the rest of their lives. They are repeat visitors to PICU, not only with whatever underlying condition they have, but also with newly acquired conditions to which they are now susceptible:

pneumonia, infections, flu and RSV (respiratory syncytial virus). And now with COVID-19.

Jason was completely fit and well before this. His body is strong from sport, athletics and basketball. But there is a sense of inevitability to his having ended up here. His life is not at all easy. It is an oversimplification to suggest that poverty alone led him here. But social determinants of health have never been more important. The list of precursors to risk is never-ending, but includes family income, housing, gender, race, education, access to services, and adverse childhood experiences. That Jason is a black boy from a particularly deprived estate in London means that he is predestined to be more likely to suffer certain diseases, illnesses and violent crimes.

Racism is a public health emergency. And it's endemic in the NHS, too. Black, Asian and minority ethnic staff are lower paid, and almost a third have experienced bullying and harassment by colleagues, according to the NHS workforce race equality data. The racial inequalities in people dying from COVID-19 – black people are four times more likely to die than white people – are devastatingly predictable. And therefore preventable. Government cutbacks have removed vital support for children like Jason. It should be shocking that a fifteen-year-old – a child – has been repeatedly stabbed with a kitchen knife, but it's not. Nurses, doctors and allied health professionals working in cities on trauma units see injuries from machete attacks, which I can't even bear to think about. Jason's injuries look minor in comparison to some of those that the UK increasingly witnesses. But stab wounds can be misleading. The wound may look small, a slit on a coin machine, yet the hidden injuries can be devastating.

Jason has three small slits in his pelvis. He's being monitored in the high-dependency area when he suddenly deteriorates. He stops shouting and his face changes shape. It's a scary thing, trauma. The compensatory mechanisms that usually enable people – children particularly – to maintain homeostasis (a stable equilibrium) for a long time and retain their blood pressure do not apply with stabbings. People fall rapidly – literally and metaphorically. They are there, present. And then they are not.

He stops swearing and thrashing around and becomes very quiet. The numbers on his monitor begin to change and cause alarm. His face suddenly looks much younger. Jason's a handsome boy. Beautiful almost, with high cheekbones and perfect skin. His eyes glaze over and his face looks shocked, as if he's realising this could be bad – worse than he thought. As if he's realising he might die.

The nurses scurry around him. There's a student nurse holding a bag of fluid next to his bed, pushing it into his vein, squeezing the bag: there's no time to put the fluid through a device that regulates its speed. Another nurse is moving furniture (always a bad sign), pushing the yellow waste bin out of the way, and wheeling in a crash trolley. Jason is losing blood. His blood pressure is falling, his heart rate increasing. The consultant, rushes over, examines his abdomen, presses softly. Jason cries out. His belly is shiny, swelling up, filling with blood. Where he's bleeding from remains a mystery.

We can see, though, that he's bleeding to death internally, even if only through subtle signs. 'Get him to theatre – we can't stabilise him here.' The consultant is a quick decision-maker. We put an oxygen cylinder on the bed, get the kit ready. I draw up cardiac-arrest drugs and put them in a small cardboard tray, ready to go. A colleague phones the blood bank to flag up that Jason will need a lot: eight units at least, as opposed to the one that you get during a standard blood transfusion. The protocol for a massive haemorrhage.

Jason looks very alone. None of his so-called friends have tried to visit or even call. His knuckles change colour as he clutches the sheet in pain and holds his rolled-up cut-off T-shirt. Semi-conscious, he looks terrified and much, much younger. I watch as the porter, consultant and student nurse quickly wheel him out of the unit to theatre.

I search Jason's paperwork for his family's contact details. There's no number for his mum, but there is one for his pupil referral unit, which will probably be on school holidays.

Luckily, someone answers the phone. The school nurse, Lola. There is no time to ask why she is working in August, but I'm guessing there is much to do outside school hours, and Lola takes a deep sigh as if she was expecting this call, sooner or later. 'I'll let his social worker know. And his mum.'

An hour or so after Jason is back from theatre, a woman runs in. She's carrying a basketball. She sits on the edge of Jason's bed and strokes his face. 'Been in the wars?' She glances at me, a flash of recognition that he's received life-changing injuries. She can see his drains, and I see her eyes sweep over his pelvis: the three dressings where he was stabbed. She holds up his basketball. 'Basketball player,' she says to me. And I think of the injury to Jason's pelvis, urethra and liver, and wonder if he'll play basketball again. If he'll even be continent. But Jason's face relaxes when he sees her. And he begins to cry. She holds him to her and rocks him. I close the curtains and leave them a while.

'His mum is lovely,' I whisper to the nurse in charge.

But I find out that's Lola. His school nurse.

Later his mum arrives, a broken woman, seemingly almost resigned to the idea that this has happened. She is catatonic with grief. She sits holding Jason's hand and looking at the monitors. It's unbearable to watch her. If he seemed alone before, then she seems even more alone now. It's amazing how alone someone can be in a room full of people.

'I can't lose him,' she whispers. 'Don't leave me,' she says. She cries and puts her head on Jason's pillow, right next to his. 'Don't leave me.' Then she lifts her head and looks at the monitors again, and then at me. 'Why did this happen? He's my son. My son.'

I have no words at all. So I don't say anything.

Later, on the way to collect a piece of equipment from another ward, I find Lola crying in the corridor, looking as broken as Jason's mum. 'He loves his mum. And she loves him. But I might be the only person he's ever trusted,' Lola says. 'And believe me, gaining that trust was not easy.'

Historically, school nursing was designed as a public-health measure within the NHS to address communicable diseases, inadequate nutrition in children, poor hygiene and other physical ailments that prevented children from attending school. And maybe that's not far off where school nursing is now. I remember nothing at all about my school nurse, and probably only saw her about nits or BCG vaccinations. But school nursing has now evolved into a highly advanced profession. School nurses are public-health nurses working with the primary aim of improving the health and well-being of children between the ages of five and nineteen. Their role is incredibly complex and varied. It involves all the jobs you'd imagine – delivering immunisation programmes for HPV (human papillomavirus), flu and meningitis, and emergency first aid – but much more besides. School nurses provide health promotion and act as a link between families, schools and children, as well as supporting individual families whose children have complex health needs and/or disabilities. They lead in the development of research-based programmes to deliver care to a diverse population of students, promoting autonomy, dignity, privacy and human rights. Mostly, though, the school nurse's job nowadays is about mental health and child protection. School nurses are the first healthcare point of call (sometimes the only point of call) for vulnerable young people like Jason. And, like all nursing, school nursing is political.

'If these were white, middle-class kids dying on the streets, knife crime would be at the top of everyone's political agenda,' Lola tells me later, and I agree with her.

The cost of a life. I think of Jason's living situation, housing and education, and of the social-care cutbacks that will have affected them. I think of his possible futures, and everything that could go wrong for him: the prospect of prison and the lack of homeless shelters, and the chance that he'll abuse substances, but not find a mental-health bed or team if – and when – he becomes seriously unwell. I imagine any one of us living his life, and how we would probably have a knife in our backpack, too. I think of all the black boys who are killed by overt or covert racism in our society. I imagine my son's future, growing up in our society in the care system.

What that future might look like for him. How much goodness he holds. How good Jason might have been. I am angry and scared for my son. Terrified.

But none of this anger helps Jason. Because he dies during the night.

I am cleaning his bed space the next day when I find out. I wash down the bed and equipment, and find the basketball in his bedside cupboard. Finally I wipe Jason's name from the board above the bed space. My stomach hurts. I don't know what to do with the basketball, so find the notes and call Lola.

She's crying quietly, but her voice is not at all shocked. 'Hurt people hurt people,' she says. 'He just needed help. Help that wasn't there. His youth centre was closed, his pupil referral unit is struggling to get teaching staff, his social worker is on stress leave. I now cover four schools. I didn't have the time he needed.' Finally she sobs – a hopeless sob from deep inside her. 'His mum didn't get the support she needed.'

'I'm so sorry, Lola. I know you took the rucksack back, but I still have his basketball. Can you use it at the PRU? Or I know it's come from his school, but shall I get it to his mum?'

'Can you donate it to the hospital play team?' she says. 'I think Jason would have wanted that.' She sighs. And clicks the phone off.

And I find the saddest thing I have to do in a long time is take a basketball to the hospital play specialist and hand it over to her. 'Donated,' I say.

By a basketball player who never had a single chance.

9

Fuck off, Janet

The day I bring my son home it is my birthday. Deepa asks if I'd like to change days and I laugh out loud. I am desperate to hold him, smell him, kiss him. It has been a strange limbo time of knowing he's out there, not with me, but somehow for ever connected to me. One night I dream about an umbilical cord that stretches the length of the country, and I awake with pains in my abdomen.

We have a process of adjustment, of getting to know him, his routines, and gradually introducing him to his sister. Of course it is impossible to be gradual with this sister of his. She runs right over to him and tries to lift him – he's heavy at two – and he laughs and she laughs. And they both fall on the ground and roll about giddy. I don't get a look-in.

I have been told that he hates water. The first evening home I put them in a bubble bath and they spend half an hour making Father Christmas beards and shouting 'Ho-ho-ho!' My daughter washes his hair, and he lets her, the soap streaming down his smiling face as she tips a cup of water over him. It will be all right, I think to myself. But we are warned about a honeymoon period, and things do get very hard, very quickly.

He begins to get frightened. I am not sure what it is that scares him so much, but as the days become weeks, he almost seems to see things that aren't there and hear loud noises in his head. He travels to a different world. After the initial few days, my son spends the first six months clinging to me, clutching my arm as if his life depends on it, his fingers digging into my flesh so hard that he once draws blood. I try and carry on as normal for my daughter, who is only four, as well as for him, but it's exhausting. I begin to wonder if I've done the right thing for my daughter and for him. And this is permanent. I know that trauma manifests itself in many ways, but my son gives me no eye contact, and he flaps his arms and screams and has rages that look like seizures, eyes rolling into the back of his head. I carry on. He starts to walk – on tiptoes – and flaps his arms continuously. He lines up all his cars in a row and stares, and daytime-sleeps for hours on end. And he hoards food – I once find a biscuit in his curls. He never displayed any of these behaviours before and I wonder if he is neurodiverse, or if he just doesn't like me or want me to be his mum.

My daughter starts primary school and the first day goes well, but by day two she's had enough and screams as loudly as he does. Defiant and stubborn as ever, she decides that she'd rather be home-schooled. On day two of school she holds my leg, arms looped around my thigh, and I drag her, screaming, to the school gate, while pushing my son, who is still in his night-time Babygro in the buggy. There's a plate of dry toast tucked into the tray beneath the buggy, and I grab a piece and put it in his hand. He looks at me as if he wants eggs or porridge instead, or maybe to get dressed, and the other mums look at me, too. My son, perhaps sensing my exhaustion or embarrassment, begins to scream too. I look at my children: neither of them properly dressed, both covered in toast crumbs and tears and snot, and red-faced, clench-fisted. Eventually I join in, and the three of us screaming clears the playground as if there's a bomb scare.

This continues for a while. The screaming, and the dry toast, and the not managing to get dressed. And, in my children's case, the rage.

My mum is staying for a few days and we sit in my son's bedroom, watching him sleep in the cot bed. He makes a growling noise like a lion and, despite the social workers' advice that I keep him in our bedroom for the first six months to promote attachment, I only last three days. 'He sounds like a wild animal,' I say, telling my mum all of this. 'But what about attachment?' And then I begin to cry.

She holds me close. She smells as she always does – of fabric conditioner and chewing gum – and her arms around me make me feel safe, as they always do, despite the fact that I'm a grown woman. My own arms feel useless, unable to keep my son safe.

'I'm a failure,' I say. 'I mean, you kept me and my brother wrapped in a blanket until we were ten, and you breastfed us until we were practically teenagers. Which explains a lot of psychological damage, by the way.'

We both laugh. And the crying stops, just like that. 'I did not! And I wasn't perfect,' says my mum. 'No parent is. You're a brilliant mum.' She tries to reassure me, but I feel like a child – unsure, lacking in confidence and ability.

'I'm nothing like you. I gave them a crisp sandwich for dinner yesterday. White bread.'

She smiles, hugs me closer. 'I bet they loved that.'

My son's bedroom is small and covered in what I thought he would like, before he came home to me: dinosaurs, cars, a wooden garage, stars and planets on the wall.

He doesn't seem to like any of it. Instead he spends his time in my daughter's room, the pair of them as thick as thieves already: she plasters stolen make-up from the bathroom onto his face, or makes him watch her sing off-key into a plastic microphone, with him clapping at the end. She writes his name in Sharpie on every piece of furniture in the house and – despite the fact that he can't hold a pen, let alone write – blames it on him. 'Why would I write someone else's name, for goodness sake?' She stares right at me as if she has won.

Once, I hear her shout, 'Cardiac arrest: stand clear', and I run up the stairs two at a time to find her performing chest compressions on his abdomen so effectively that he projectile-vomits and it takes me two hours to clean it from his hair, the walls and the ceiling, before I can sit them down and explain how dangerous that is. Still, he sticks to her like she's covered in glue. And she loves him – as I do – like the world has never seen love.

But he hasn't yet attached to me. 'What if I'm wrong for him?' I whisper, looking at my son. His face is far away in a dream, moving from smiling to frowning, to surprise. His expressive face. He growls his lion growl and we laugh again.

'Do you love him?' my mum asks, as if she can read my thoughts about my daughter. Maybe she can. I can hear my daughter's thoughts in my head all the time.

'So much,' I say. I lean my head on her shoulder. 'I can't even describe it.'

She kisses the top of my head as if I am a child. 'Then it will all fall into place. I promise.'

The following week I take my daughter to her regular swimming lesson, and the noise of the leisure centre freaks my son out so much that he bites me, hard. I yelp. A woman I recognise from the local cafe where she works, who has a daughter about the same age as mine though they must go to different schools, shouts across the swimming-pool viewing area, 'Is that the adopted one?' And my son turns and listens, and I know – I absolutely know in my bones – that he understands what she has said. His face fills with tears. He is different. He does not belong. My son and I look at each other. Eye contact at last. Something shifts. 'Is that the adopted one?' she shouts over again. 'I see you are struggling.'

And I look at my son, this virtual stranger. And he looks at me, this virtual stranger. And I stand up and hold him to my body. I walk up the stairs to the exit. We walk past her, and she touches him. Actually touches him. Reaches out to touch the skin on his leg. I feel him flinch. I flinch.

I hold him closer still, with my arm around his head, away from her. And I feel his fear through my skin. And this time my arms feel stronger. I lift my head high and stare at her. And I am not my mum. I'll never be as soft as she was. Or as kind, as tolerant. But maybe that's not the kind of mum he needs anyway. I am his mum. And I love him. And everything else will fall into place.

'Oh, fuck off, Janet,' I say. And we go. And he relaxes. And for the first time he puts his head down gently on my shoulder. He rests it so gently I can barely breathe. And I kiss his head. And he lets me. And in that single moment, whatever happens, he somehow knows he is okay. We both are. And just like that, he talks and walks and laughs, and plays and runs and jumps and looks straight into my eyes. In fact every time he does anything, he glances up, to make sure I am watching. To make sure I am there.

Life after that is, for a while, pretty perfect. For the next few years, in fact. I delight in my children, in their playing, in his sudden settling, in the moments that take my breath away. I play constant peekaboo with my son, disappearing and then coming back, over and over again. Each time his confidence is growing. He is so much a part of me that once, when discussing childbirth, a woman asks about my experiences. I tell her how normal and horrific my daughter's birth was and, when she asks about my son, I pause and try to think. And it takes around ten seconds for me to remember and say that I didn't give birth to him at all.

I've always thought of all intensive cares as a kind of womb: the rhythmic noises, the controlled softness, the complete surrender of patients to the lifeline of ventilators. And the patients are babies *in utero* for a while, not quite alive but still living; and whatever happens, they will emerge different for ever, from this mother ship, the starship of another place.

It is September and I'm here as a student, even though I've been qualified for years, because this is an advanced intensive-care training course that takes me on placements, and in and out of the university, over the course of six months. This specialist training is a tough course. Critical-care nursing, like all nursing, is safety-critical and requires a high level of skill, expertise, compassion, leadership and training, and I love the studying. September is my favourite month: I always did love it, going back to school, even as a wayward teen – new note-books, expanding worlds, the crisp smell of autumn air and new possibilities, the chance to change. Going back to school throughout my nursing career, for short courses and longer ones, has sometimes meant that every month feels like September.

There is a calm about intensive care, even in the most desperate of circumstances, even on the busiest of days. And when it is impossible to save a patient, despite everyone's best efforts, the critical care nurses are able to offer dignity, a pain-free death and, perhaps most importantly, compassionate care for patients and for families. They take away what suffering they can and make sure that no one dies alone even when a family can't get to critical care in time. Critical care nurses will be with loved ones to their dying breaths, when families can't be there.

Gwen's family will not get here in time. A nurse I'm shad-owing, named Stella, sent local police to knock on the door and deliver the news that the family needs to get to the hospital as quickly as possible; and the police have offered to drive them, making sure they don't end up crashing the car on their way. Delivering bad news requires a skill and experience that is hard to describe. There is no formula. No learning can prepare you for it. Stella tries to judge a person's life – how they understand the world, what kind of beliefs or wishes they have – all based on a short conversation with a stranger.

'Gwen's son, David, told me that his dad, Bill, is also with him, but he can't speak. He's crying too much.' Stella sighs. She's been an intensive-care nurse for thirty-one years. It doesn't get any easier. 'Imagine them sitting there, in the back of a police car, with David trying to explain to his dad that his mum is seriously ill on a ventilator and might die. Terrible thing sometimes, this life.' She looks across the ward at Gwen.

Gwen is wearing a hospital gown and is decorated with tubes and lines and wires: an endotracheal tube, a central venous line and arterial line, a vascath and nasogastric tube, ECG dots, defib pads, IV cannulas. There's hardly any way to identify her underneath all the equipment and machinery keeping her alive, but I notice her bitten fingernails, her thick gold wedding ring, her dark-brown hair. I see a small tattoo of a bumble bee on her shoulder. Later I will learn that she and Bill, her husband, were beekeepers. These are the details that make us human, and they are what intensive-care nurses do their best to remember. We are more than our illnesses, our hospitalisation.

Gwen is only sixty-one, but has COPD – chronic obstructive pulmonary disease – and has developed pneumonia, which is proving to be resistant to antibiotics. Antibiotic resistance terrifies me. I've cared for patients who have started out with relatively minor injuries, yet have developed bacterial infections that are resistant to treatment, or even untreatable. And then a small wound becomes necrotic, or gangrenous. A body eating itself, while we can only keep trying new drugs. Bacteria and fungi and viruses are fascinating and clever: nature's nuclear weapons. Whenever I see reports that – understandably – panic about climate change and the possibility of the extinction of humanity, I hear my nurse-heart whisper, *What about antibiotic-resistant bacteria?* And then along comes, instead of bacteria, a virus: COVID-19.

Gwen has developed ARDS (acute respiratory distress syndrome), a serious lung condition causing respiratory failure, something known in intensive care as 'wet lungs'. The membranes that keep fluid out of the tissues in the lungs break down, causing the bases of the lungs to leak and flood and, if not treated, effectively drown the patient. The aim of treatment with a ventilator is to give patients like Gwen a high PEEP, which by keeping the lungs open with pressure forces more room into them for oxygen exchange. It's a bit like blowing up a balloon. The first part of the blowing is the hardest – and PEEP via a ventilator avoids that first exhausting part by keeping the balloon from collapsing between each breath. ARDS is always life-threatening. For those who do survive, their life is often changed for ever. For example, someone may have long-term brain, kidney and lung damage. They may never go back to work.

We are going to be hearing a lot more about ARDS. COVID-19 causes death by heart failure and multi-organ failure, preceded by pneumonitis that is similar to ARDS and can develop into ARDS itself, which fills the lungs with fluid and kills around 50 per cent of coronavirus patients who get it. As for the other 50 per cent – the survivors of this complication – the outcome remains to be seen. Survival, I suspect, for all of us is only the beginning. How will we all live with the knowledge that our loved ones died such a terrible death? And, even worse, the possibility that the most precious members of our families died without us by their side?

But there is always compassion.

There is always hope.

When Gwen's heart stops, Stella is immediately on her chest, pressing down, as if her body is on a tight coil, pulled into action in a split second. Another nurse wheels the crash trolley over. In critical care, the crash trolley is always perfect, but I've been to other areas of the hospital and seen all sorts of things. The items that I find on crash trolleys, in addition to out-of-date drugs or banned, unsafe equipment, are always surprising: a vase full of knitting needles, which had me imagining injury all day, with an over-enthusiastic junior anaesthetist maybe thinking they were airway tools of some sort; a pocket book of Shakespeare's Sonnets; a jar of pickled gherkins.

The team are around Gwen in a flash and doing everything in their power to save her. I act as scribe, writing down everything: the drugs, the timings of shocks, the cardiac-arrest rhythms. Gwen is the sickest patient on the unit. It takes seven members of staff to manage her resuscitation, and I am certain she will not survive it. I keep looking at the door. Her husband will surely appear any minute and see his beloved wife slipping away from this world, despite our best efforts.

But I also hear a voice from long ago in my head: *Faith is not knowing. It's hoping.*

A nurse takes over from Stella after the first two-minute cycle. Chest compressions are exhausting. Stella comes to catch her breath next to me, then takes over the defibrillator. After another round we pause, check the defib, and there is a squiggly line as if a child has drawn it, which is a shockable cardiac-arrest rhythm and what gives you the most chance of survival. Stella charges the machine, shouts orders to stand clear, presses the button to shock and then gets everyone back on Gwen's chest, and back to work.

Somehow, Gwen survives. The team are relieved, delighted – they know her family are en route. When Gwen's son David rushes in, she has stabilised and his panicked eyes can see that she is still here, still alive, even if only just.

I watch Bill walk over to his wife, and I pull the curtains slightly so that they can have some privacy. We don't know if Gwen will make it. Probably not. But Bill will always know that he was with her, right next to her, holding her hand.

And in that moment, there is only them. A husband and his wife.

Bill leans over and kisses Gwen as if she doesn't have a single tube or wire anywhere. He kisses her as if he might never get the chance again.

10

The Golden Hour

It's a cruel, strange truth that all too often everything bad happens at once. Crying is another funny thing. You can feel as if you have no more tears anywhere inside you, yet they keep coming, as if you contain an entire river. I cry so hard my lips are dry; I must be dehydrated, but they keep coming. My children – my son, aged five, and my daughter, seven – are crying too. They cry and cry and cry. And every time I look at them, I feel like the worst mum in the world, the biggest failure.

The day we move out of our family home and into a small rented house I try and suppress the crying. We have two burly removal men, paid for with the very last money I have. I am writing and nursing and teaching and planning to work ninety-hour weeks, helped by a live-in au pair staying in a boxroom. I am not sure how we will pay the extortionate London rent, but I will make it work – I must. I don't want to move the children from school and nursery, not now. Besides, we have nowhere else to go. The removal men stop their whistling and cheerful chat as soon as they turn up. They find me sitting among the half-packed-up boxes, my children wailing beside me. They want their dad. They want us not to split up. They want to stay in their house. But we can't afford to. And I have no way of comforting them. No words, no energy – nothing. I am empty of everything but tears.

The day of my paternal granddad's funeral, my brother and I drive up to Lincolnshire and we stop at a restaurant. My dad is dying – we don't know this yet, but he will die next week. All we know is how frail and ill he is, and how desperately sad he is that he can't go to his own father's funeral. What a thing, we think, not to be able to go to a loved one's funeral. Somehow my brother and I still manage to crack a joke. A smile. A sarcastic comment. That family gallows-humour. But it doesn't do much to cover our pain. We order food, which we don't eat, and talk about how long our dad might have left.

My brother, who is the fittest person I know, starts to feel unwell. This is unusual. He loves to tell people that, as well as being Italian (we're not), he is pretty much an Olympic athlete, as his resting heart rate is forty-five. He is the strongest and healthiest person I know. And despite his jokey bragging – I once heard him say he'd basically invented Ibiza – he's also the best of men. But he begins sweating and looks pale. 'I'll get some air,' he says and steps out of the restaurant. And everything slows down a bit, time seeming to stop and freeze. I watch him.

There are floor-to-ceiling windows. I look at my brother outside and the slow-motion sensation gets worse. He is staggering in the near-empty street, with its cobbled stones and neat, pretty houses opposite. But we are not drinking. And we are a million years from the drug-taking of our adolescence. I think perhaps he is joking around, and I take a small sip of soup. And he is leaning forward. I smile, but something about his face isn't right. He's not smiling, not even with his eyes, as he always is. And then, just like that, he falls. He falls.

My soup spoon drops to the floor as well, clanging, and there is an utter, unbearable silence. For a few seconds I'm unable to move. I can't breathe. Not him. Not my brother. Every man in my life has fallen away. Except him. I am not religious, but I want to scream at the sky: *What more do you want from me?* Instead I run. I shove open the door and rush over to him. By the time I'm outside, a small crowd has gathered. Someone has phoned for an ambulance. And he is on the ground, not responding. And there are flashing lights. And his eyes are shut. And, and, and ...

It's a long time before I feel lucky. I walk over the bridge towards the hospital. My footsteps land in the same place, yet everything feels different. There have always been homeless people on this bridge, or dotted around the hospital in stairwells and shadows, searching for sanctuary. And yet now there are pop-up tents everywhere – entire communities of rough sleepers lining the road. The Houses of Parliament are nearby and must have the same view: of our homeless city, of the people barely surviving, their fingers ulcerated and swollen and their clothes soiled, hair matted.

As I walk towards the hospital a man lies semi-conscious with his trousers half down, exposed. He has vomit near his head. I watch people walk past him. How invisible he seems. I stop and shake him gently, but although he moans, he doesn't wake properly. He is out of it, with some substance or other – as we all might be, in the same circumstances, I suspect. 'Hello, can you hear me?' He cracks open one eye. I can tell he's breathing normally. More people walk past: a woman wearing heels; men in suits; hospital workers; doctors and nurses, too. All on phones, texting as they walk. I kneel beside this man and feel such despair. I have no idea who he is, I have no connection to him, and yet to be exposed and vulnerable and to have people side-stepping – almost walking over – his body makes me feel rage.

I watch the river below us. The sun is rising, making golden patterns on the dancing water. This river that must have seen so much. A friend from the Democratic Republic of the Congo tells me that 'Congo' means the 'River that Swallows All Stories'. I think the Thames, too, must have swallowed all stories, and seen life improve for so many and then get worse again. We are tidal and nothing really changes; life simply moves continuously forward and backwards. And now is the backwards moment, it seems: Dickens's London once more.

Almost one in fifty Londoners are homeless. And this is pre COVID-19.

But that's not so everywhere. In Dundee I meet plenty of homeless people, yet not one of them is sleeping rough. 'About five rough sleepers in the city,' a woman tells me. 'The rest of us have shelters or short-term accommodation.' I travel to other towns and cities in Scotland and find a similar story. 'I come to the soup kitchen every Wednesday,' a Scottish housing worker tells me. 'Sit and help however I can.' She explains that there is virtually no rough sleeping in Scotland because people are not told they need to prove that they are homeless before being offered accommodation. 'In England, people need to prove it,' she says. 'And I don't know many people who carry documents when they are in crisis.'

Perhaps that is why we see so many people sleeping rough in England? According to Shelter, homelessness is defined as anyone experiencing the following situations: no accommodation available in the UK or abroad; no legal right to occupy accommodation; split households and the unavailability of accommodation for a whole household; it is deemed unreasonable to continue to occupy accommodation; there is the probability of violence; the applicant is unable to secure entry to accommodation or lives in a moveable structure, but has no place to put this. This encompasses rough sleepers, but essentially means anyone who has no fixed address or is at risk of homelessness.

Regardless of the way in which someone is defined as homeless, all over the UK teams of nurses support the health of people who are living without a home. And that support is desperately, and increasingly, needed. The homeless charity Crisis reports that people sleeping on the street are almost seventeen times more likely to have been the victims of violence. More than one in three people sleeping rough have been deliberately hit or kicked, or have experienced some other form of violence while homeless. The average life expectancy of a homeless person is just forty-four years old. A Queen's Nurse working with a Community Mental Health Team that covers five hostels and several hundred temporary furnished homeless flats, describes her work as 'caring for social problems as well as health and well-being'. She clearly loves her job. Of her clients, she says, 'I get to meet some of the most courageous and brave individuals. It's an honour.'

I keep her words in my head and pull the man's trousers up as best I can and his sleeping bag over him, for it is already getting cold. Gearing up for winter in the NHS means knowing that people will die from the cold. Rough sleepers will freeze to death. A woman once describes how it feels to me, to freeze. She had been admitted to A&E, hypothermic after sleeping outside. She survived somehow, but it was winter and minus five degrees. 'Freezing felt like burning,' she tells me. 'As if my skin was on fire. It was the worst pain I ever felt – the cold.

I tried to scream, but I couldn't move. And I can't remember anything after that.'

As I walk towards the hospital, I do not look back at Parliament. It's more important that they look out of the windows than that we look in.

A&E is stupidly busy. It's chaos. It is October and this doesn't bode well. October is the start of the busy period, but it's only early in the month and we are a long way from the quieter spring. Yet already corridors are lined with patients on trolleys; there are patients and relatives, and a man is screaming from a cubicle. I walk past a woman who is sitting behind a cloud of nebuliser, a crossword puzzle on her lap. She waves as I walk past. I wave back. The next bed has curtains around it, but I can hear laughing behind the curtains. A porter runs past, nearly knocking me out of the way, and I navigate my way around a cleaner who is polishing the floor with a large electric machine.

In the next cubicle a man is making constant cycling movements in the air, as though he is riding an invisible bike. His breathing is exaggerated and deep, and is following a strange pattern: a stroke. There is no good time or place to have a stroke, but this hospital does not have a hyper-acute stroke unit and so he'll probably need transferring: within ninety minutes, if his brain on fire is to be meaningfully preserved. This may seem a long time, but time flies by in hospitals. A younger woman sits next to him – his daughter perhaps – and her face is somewhere else with worry. Maybe in the future, or maybe in the past: what if; or what could be. Life is so random. A stroke often comes from nowhere and changes a person's entire life. I look away.

My friend dies of a stroke while I am writing this book. And I find it hard to look at any male patient in his sixties without thinking of my own dad, and the image I can't shake is of his dying body: the expression on his face as he took his last breath; the expression on my mum's face. Grief is always fresh; time never heals. I've learned this the hard way. There is no quick fix, no perfect recovery. You live with it. And some days are harder than others, no matter how long ago the loss happened.

Nurses and doctors and other healthcare professionals must all find it hard to escape the recent painful memories of a loved one dying and get back to memories of a happier time, because there is pain and death in front of us every day. But there's always something to shock us out of our own thoughts, too. Being busy helps. Having no time to think or process emotion is a strange (albeit probably unhealthy) comfort. And A&E never fails to remind me that there is always someone, somewhere, suffering something worse.

A woman in the next cubicle is hooked up to a blood transfusion, wrapped in many blankets, yet her bones are still sharp beneath them, her hair wispy and patchy. A&E is no place for cancer patients. But it's often where people suffering from all manner of cancers are initially diagnosed, having been rushed in with complications or in severe pain. In the next bed a heroin user has overdosed, and the nurse is pushing Narcan, the antidote, into a precious venous line. The nurse jumps out of the way as soon as the drug is administered, which, in my experience, is the right thing to do. People can wake up suddenly and violently, and it's not unheard of for patients to lash out as they wake. Nurses routinely give out Narcan to communities of substance-misusers in case one of them has an overdose, and they treat each other. This simple initiative has saved countless lives. The simple things often make the most difference.

I walk past and hear a mature student nurse introduce herself to a patient with a guide dog and then ask the patient, 'What's your name? And how do you like to be known? Oh, what a lovely dog!' And it makes me smile, thankful that some things are moving in a good direction. I remember the days when the idea of asking what pronoun a patient preferred would have been laughed out of the room, by both the nurse and the probably confused patient. Student nurses these days teach me a lot about language and respect and progress.

Sandra, the sister, bustles past covered in two aprons with a visor-type plastic mask on her head and a theatre mask hanging round her neck. 'Can you help log-roll?' There are nurses I've worked with in the past who like to look busy continuously, even when they're not. Sandra is not one of them. She doesn't stop. She's constantly got a swarm of people around her asking for different things, both nurses and doctors. Watching her at work is like watching the conductor of an orchestra. A&E has a strange music. All hospital departments have their own beats and melodies and, if you listen carefully enough, you can hear them and work out what kind of shift it will be. It is a soundtrack in the heads of the staff, and probably the patients, too. I've started to notice correlations between different hospital areas and music – plus art. While A&E, like the mental-health unit, has a print on the wall of Monet's *Water Lilies*, it is really more of an abstract painting, maybe Jackson Pollock.

Sandra's footsteps are part of the A&E music: angry steps, the early squeak of her nurse's shoes long since gone, now a loud and steady – almost relentless – pace. 'Wendy is a known rough sleeper,' she tells me. 'Some little bastards have attacked her.' Sandra dries her hands with a scratchy NHS hand-towel. 'This world we live in.' But she does not seem surprised. Total and utter cruelty is on the rise in our society, and those on the margins have somehow become targets: people with disabilities, the LGBT+ community, the homeless, black people and those from minority ethnic communities. A&E staff are dealing with hate-crime at unprecedented levels. I ask Sandra why there seems to be increasing pain and anger nowadays. Why so many people feel such hatred. 'The question is why people suffer, not why they hate. Because, underneath all that hatred, there is so much fear in our world. I'd still like to kill the little bastards, though. We had a homeless man in last week who had been set on fire, and a ten-year-old bullied for being gay,' she continues. 'He ran out in front of a bus.' Sandra has seen everything the world has to offer.

Wendy is a bloody mess when I meet her. Her face looks like it's been through a mincer: her nose is half hanging off; she's clearly suffered fractures to the bones around her eyes; one of her eyes looks displaced, sunken, and there are huge black rings around both of them, while the sclera – the whites of her eyes – are blood-red. She's wearing a spinal collar and, in the absence of sandbags, has two bags of fluid and towels rolled up next to her face, taped across her forehead and chin to keep her neck still. Her T-shirt has been cut open, and I can see a large healed cardiac scar down the centre of her chest; and there are patches of bruises, the colour of oil slicks, all down her abdomen and right side. Her left leg is at an odd angle and her right leg looks shorter. Her trousers are ripped to shreds.

I watch the police officers gathered at the nurses' station. They are in A&E all the time. Many doctors I know hate the term 'Accident and Emergency', preferring 'Emergency Department', perhaps because so much of their work is about life-threatening injuries that are not at all 'accidental'. I can't imagine what kind of person could do this to another human being: beating and kicking and hurting them. And why the number of people treated in such a way is increasing so dramatically. Politics has always been part of nursing, but our current political situation means a rise of hatred, and it seeps into healthcare like poison into water.

'Ready to log-roll, folks?' Sandra is at the head end – that's the important bit. A log-roll is exactly what it sounds like: rolling a person as if they are a log, moving their body as little as possible because they have a suspected (or actual) injury to their C-spine. It takes four people: Sandra is holding Wendy's head and neck completely still; a doctor is standing next to me; a nurse is waiting behind us to pull out the board that Wendy is lying on; and I'm near her feet. I'm always at that end, because we stand in height order, and I'm short. Sandra explains to Wendy what is happening and then makes eye contact with all of us, before telling us clearly what she will do and how she will communicate: 'On "move",' she says. We try and avoid 'One, two, three' because people never know if it's on three or after three, and unless we move in complete unison Wendy's spine is at risk.

'Ready, steady, move.'

We roll Wendy towards us and the nurse pulls out the hard board from the trolley and carefully inspects Wendy's back, running her fingers down her spine as though she is playing a piano. Wendy is sleepy, having had strong pain medication, but groans a bit. We roll her back, again on a command, and the assessment is complete. She'll be reassessed again when she's fully awake.

The crash bell goes off almost immediately, and everyone scatters like leaves in the wind. I lean out of the curtains and can see that the cycling man across the ward has stopped cycling. He has a team around him within seconds, all performing different jobs. A mask is being pressed over his nose and mouth. He must have stopped breathing. His daughter is standing at the bottom of his bed with her hand over her mouth. I feel as though I've been punched in the stomach. As though I'm watching myself, or any daughter who has lost her dad.

I pull the curtains back round. Take a breath. Sandra is washing her hands. She turns. 'There's enough of them out there,' she says to Wendy. 'Let's me and Christie get you washed up a bit.'

Sandra opens a pack of sterile gloves and lays out some saline, gauze and dressings. She carefully starts to wash and dress Wendy's wounds, working from head to toe on one side, while I mirror her on the other side. I clean and steri-strip the cuts above Wendy's eye and, as I do so, she begins to wake and focus a bit more.

'Wendy, we're in hospital. We're helping you. My name is Sandra.' I watch Sandra talk with her hands, voice and eyes. Communication is, for the most part, not about words. It does not surprise me to find out that Sandra has, in her own time, learned Makaton, a language designed to help hearing people who have learning or communication difficulties to communicate. Like many nurses, she might as well have 'Badass' written on her name badge. Her face is hard at the edges, her humour sharp and she is as tough as they come. But she has advanced clinical skills and is so, so compassionate. 'Your key worker, Clara, is coming in, but one of us nurses will stay with you until then. Try to keep still and relax. I know it's scary, but I'm right here.'

We manage to clean most of the blood from Wendy's skin, and Sandra administers some IV pain medication and records all of Wendy's observations: her blood pressure, temperature, respiratory rate and heart rate, as well as the oxygen level in her blood via a SaO2 machine that uses a red laser light on a fingertip. I notice that Wendy has clubbing of her fingers – bulbous, round ends and flat nailbeds – that might be cardiac-related. Sandra calls to a healthcare assistant to sit with Wendy for a while for, despite her having fallen asleep, until her C-spine is properly cleared, there is real danger if she wakes and tries to move suddenly.

We walk towards the nurses' station so that Sandra can talk to the police. 'I'll refer her to the safeguarding team, too, and get advice about sexual assault. It's a possibility.'

My eyes burn. I don't know how Sandra does this job every day. Knowing that I can drift in and out of A&E is a comfort:

I don't feel tough enough to deal with whatever comes through the door. I wonder what drives a nurse to pick A&E as their speciality. There are nurses who get off on the adrenaline, who get excited when the red phone announces a serious trauma: a bus full of children that has crashed; a terrorist attack at Westminster; a fire on the Underground. I see their faces change at the thought of the 'golden hour' – the hour immediately after injury – that critical time period when the team can save someone's life. Every minute, every second counts. It's also a term described to me by an artist I meet at a medical humanities conference being run by Sam Guglani – a clinical oncologist and a novelist. He is searching for meaning in narrative medicine: the idea that art and story have much to offer medicine, and that they might help him and his patients make sense of this life. He understands that even the best science can only cure us sometimes. Whereas art doesn't seek to cure, but often saves us anyway. The artist shows me photos of her work. 'I only paint during the golden hour. That moment between day and night when the light is perfect. When anything seems possible. When buildings are their most beautiful and raw.'

I think about those raw, in-between times in medicine, when all other issues are nothing. There is only humanity and survival, and all that is important are family and loved ones. It is perhaps then that we emit the most perfect of human light. And it is also in those moments that, to me, nurses and doctors and all members of the multi-disciplinary team appear at their most capable, when their skills and experience all come together. They forget everything else – their focus is entirely pure. I wonder if that is what draws people to A&E: the chance to live in the golden hour.

It takes a long time to embody this understanding. As we are walking out of the unit later, we can hear singing. Sandra frowns and looks at me. She ups her pace, and as we get towards the singing there are loud voices and alarms, and a swarm of people around the bed of an elderly lady who is being resuscitated by a team of people. A medical student wearing a badge that says 'Hello, My Name is Giles (Medical Student)' is performing vigorous chest compressions and is probably breaking all the woman's ribs, although this won't matter if she survives. Covered in sweat, bright red, he is singing loudly 'Another One Bites the Dust' as he presses on the poor woman's chest.

Sandra glares at him, but he misses her point and, instead of stopping, starts singing 'Stayin' Alive'. When he sees her hands move to her hips, he clearly doesn't know what to do and switches to 'Nelly the Elephant'. Sandra almost has steam coming out of her ears. But, worse, the woman is not having a cardiac arrest at all, which should be obvious to the rest of the team, given that she is waving her arms in the air (to be fair, almost in time with Giles's singing).

Eventually Sandra physically pulls him off. I'm worried she will slap Giles across the face or something that is likely to get her up before a disciplinary board meeting, so I pull her away slightly, creating a domino effect. One of the doctors walking past surveys the scene and, quickly assessing what Sandra is dealing with, begins to laugh. Sandra gives him a look of sarcasm, slight exasperation and friendship.

The patient rolls over and starts to move her limbs and moan. Giles throws his hand over his mouth, realising his mistake.

I feel sorry for him. During my first week as a resuscitation officer I find a man who is the colour of pigeon-shit, certainly dead, slumped on a chair outside the twenty-four-hour sandwich bar where I am queuing for a tuna melt at the end of my shift. I race over, pull him to the floor by his legs and start compressing his chest and shouting for help. The man suddenly takes a large breath and tells me to get lost. He isn't dead in the slightest, just taking a nap. 'If someone can tell you to fuck off, they are probably fine,' my colleague tells me.

I smile as I remember this. Giles is doing his best, as I was.

'If a patient tries to swat you away while you're doing chest compressions,' says Sandra through her teeth, 'they are not dead.'

Giles lets his hand drop. 'I'm so sorry. I had my Immediate Life Support training last week and it must have been on my mind.'

I watch Sandra's face for a reaction. She'd be perfectly correct to explain to Giles that having chest compressions when not in cardiac arrest is painful and stressful, and likely to make the clinical picture much, much worse. But I see her frown line flatten a fraction. We've all been new to this. 'For next time, "Nelly the Elephant" is too slow,' she says. And she winks. 'And for God's sake sing in your head. This isn't *The X Factor.*'

We return to Wendy, and Sandra sits down next to her. 'I'm going to ask you a ton of questions now,' she says. 'I'd like to know about your life. It will help us to look after you, so you tell me whatever you think we need to know. What things you like to eat and drink, and all those things.'

Details are vital. I looked after a child once who was nearly given urgent treatment – strong and potentially dangerous drugs – for coning (brain stem herniation), which is a neuro-surgical emergency that means the brain is being squashed into the spinal cord. He had symptoms of a fixed dilated pupil and abnormal posture. However, this child had cerebral palsy and was blind – so he always had a fixed dilated pupil and his posture was always unusual. Luckily the nurses read the admission nurse's notes, which highlighted that this was normal for him, before he was given unnecessary or even harmful treatment.

Sandra writes *Hate-crime* on the admission paperwork. Of course the fact that Wendy is homeless makes a paperwork trail more difficult, although the nurses do their best to link up the services. Sandra discovers that Wendy is being cared for by the Homeless Health Nursing team, who see her regularly in clinic and in hostels, and when she is sleeping rough, day and night.

The cost-saving implications of the Homeless Health Nursing teams for the NHS are immense. Justine Bohan, a peripatetic nurse, led a pilot peripatetic nurse service in Hammersmith and Fulham in 2017, in which she travelled to homeless hostels and walk-in day centres for rough sleepers, providing care support and treatment. It led to a 20 per cent reduction in A&E admissions. But the real value of Homeless Health Nursing specialists is more important than money. A homeless man tells me of his nurse, 'She helps me survive. Makes me remember that I am a human being and that I deserve healthcare, same as everyone else.'

The sociology of healthcare and the politics of our time increasingly spill into NHS hospitals and clinics – but hate-crime has always been with us. When I am fifteen, my dad finds himself working long hours every day for free at the local Londis store after the owner, my dad's friend, is the victim of a racially motivated attack and has to spend months in hospital. The local kids run into the shop and shout racist slurs at my dad until he chases them out with a broom.

We are living in a time of ever-increasing division and hatred and political turmoil. And, at times, of cruelty. But remembering my dad – who, opinionated and offensive as he could be at times, was so immediately protective and compassionate towards any other human being – gives me hope. If he ever saw someone hurt another person, he would stand up against them. Sometimes he would get things wrong and cause offence, but he always stood up anyway. My dad and I disagreed about everything, yet still respected and loved each other. He taught me that it is possible to be at opposite ends of a political argument and remain good friends.

'Doesn't matter what you think. If you see another person being hurt and don't step in to help, you are as bad as the person doing the hurting.' My dad was a rogue. But he always had the courage to care.

Wendy is crying when I see her later. She's being discharged. She's covered in bandages, and she has no medical reason to be admitted to a ward. She is facing another night on the street. She is shaking with fear. 'It's like I'm not even human,' she says. 'Who would do that? It's not my fault I'm homeless. Could happen to anyone.'

I am rushing between jobs, trying to fill in the audit forms that we write following any crash calls, in order that we can monitor and improve our service. I need to head up to the cardiac wards, where a man has had seven dangerous arrhythmias in the space of a week, all needing cardioversion – a shock to the heart that flicks his electricity into a normal rhythm. I want to stay with Wendy. To hear her story. And I can see that she wants to tell me. I wonder what kind of life led her here, what her history contains, who she loves in this world and who loves her. But perhaps there is nobody.

Nursing is a busy profession. My job is complex and academic and involves time management, risk assessment and priorities. I know that the man on the cardiac ward is at risk. He might die if his cardiac arrhythmias are not properly managed, and the pattern of his medical emergencies and treatments during them is important information that must be found out, to help the team of specialists caring for him, even in a small way. Today, like many days, I've not eaten breakfast, or lunch. The A&E staff are buzzing around from one emergency to another and have probably not even drunk water, let alone eaten.

Wendy's problems are no longer medical. The NHS is full of patients waiting for desperately needed beds. It is not the job of the NHS to provide shelter or housing, or food or heating. I have no time to sit with Wendy, hold her hand and listen, no matter how much I want to. Helping people who need help is the reason many people become nurses, and all too often we can't. But nurses find ways to help sometimes, despite – not because of – the system.

Sandra comes towards us carrying a pile of medical notes so high that she's balanced them underneath her chin. 'Right then, Wendy,' she says, 'I hear Dr Afolayan said you're ready for discharge.' She puts the pile of notes down at the end of Wendy's bed. 'But, silly me, I forgot to tell him about the chest pain.'

Wendy stops crying. 'What chest pain?'

Sandra shakes her head slightly and speaks clearly and slowly. 'Well, I know you're ready for discharge, but obviously the chest pain means that we need to find you a bed to do some further tests. Especially with your cardiac history.'

There's a pause. Then Wendy smiles. 'It's quite bad,' she says and presses her hand in the centre of her chest, somewhere near her heart.

'Thought so,' says Sandra, her badass voice clipped and no-nonsense. She stands and picks up the notes, and winks at me as she walks away.

'I think I need morphine,' says Wendy, still holding her chest.

'No chance,' I say, and we grin at each other.

After many months in our new rented house, with me working ninety hours a week, and worrying and worrying and writing and writing, I am finally seeing a bigger picture. I often remember patients and their families who have been in far worse situations and have gone through far worse things. We have a roof over our head, food in the cupboards and a family who loves us. We have my brother.

We never find out what caused a man as strong as him to fall that day. The paramedics said it could be a cardiac arrhythmia or low blood sugar, but whatever it was, it passed. I perform a twelve-lead ECG on him at work – in a cupboard – to check his heart. I show a nurse colleague, an expert in ECGs, the printout and she shrugs. 'Normal. And remember it's amazing what stress can do.'

My brother smiles, lifts an arm and flexes a muscle. 'Unbreakable,' he says. And the world moves again – more slowly than before, but it moves. We are lucky.

I still feel awful guilt for my children, though, who are doing their best. They did not ask for all this. I decide on a whim to take them to a caravan park. It's October half-term and there's a cheap offer, and my mum and dad always took us on caravan holidays. Once, when my dad had been made redundant, we stayed an entire summer, my mum washing her hair in the river with washing-up liquid. I still remember how soft her hair was, the way it smelled. Life had given my parents lemons then and they made happy memories, regardless, for us kids. I want to try and be more like them. And my two are beyond excited. My son actually screams. They once went to Butlin's with my mum and dad and said it was the best place in the world. Of course, much as I'm trying to channel my mother's style of parenting, I am not my mum. And I can't imagine anything worse than a caravan holiday. But the look on the children's faces is everything and, for the first time in months, I smile properly.

It is worse than I imagined. I'm weird about food, and the buffet is coughed over by people who pile so much food onto their plates that bread rolls, hot-dog sausages and chicken legs fall to the ground and are kicked about, leaving a shiny snail trail of grease. The children, though, love it. When I tell them to have whatever they want, they look at me suspiciously, as if it's a trick.

In the evenings the worst entertainment I have ever experienced is topped off by a man in a bear costume walking around and hugging the adults as well as the children. I do not want to be hugged. But they love that, too. It's heaven for them. They make friends and are happy. I sit quietly, feeling depressed and tired, watching them and trying to find joy in their joy. The nightly show ends with the children onstage trying to win a star prize. The adults, all couples, sit at the bar area and appear to be having a good time, laughing and drinking. I can't bear to hear them. I am in two minds about getting my earplugs from the caravan, but decide to stick it out and instead order a bucket of Pinot Grigio and sit at an empty table, waving to the children. The bartender laughs when I order, thinking I am joking, but then sees my scowling face and pours the biggest glass of wine I have ever seen.

My daughter at the front of the stage is surrounded by new friends, her face painted as a butterfly. My son is onstage trying to win the prize. The giant bear is next to him. Barney – the bear – has a microphone. He asks the children in turn random stuff, such as do they like ice-cream. Then he reaches my son. 'Who are you here with?' he asks. He looks out over the bar. 'You here with Mummy and Daddy?'

And my son, beaming with pride, arms shaking with excitement at the prospect of winning some plastic tat, points over at me. The bear hands him a microphone. 'I'm with my mummy,' he says, his voice full of lisp. 'Not my daddy. Because she's getting a divorsssse.'

And a spotlight lands on my head just as I am chugging back a huge mouthful of wine.

11

Precious Scars

Rose is eighty-seven and suffering from dementia and renal failure (which we now call 'acute kidney injury') and so she has become even more confused and disorientated. Eventually she is almost catatonic.

I am living with my nan and working at the local hospital as a healthcare assistant alongside my nurse's training – I'm doing it for the money, but also for the extra experience. Healthcare assistants, sometimes called nursing assistants, are an essential skilled part of the healthcare workforce who assist with physical care, record observations and provide emotional support, along with many other things. It's a busy day and I've a number of tasks on my to-do list, including washing and dressing patients. Rose is first on that list.

I bring the curtain round and balance a bowl of warm soapy water on her bedside table. 'I'm Christie, the healthcare assistant,' I say to her. 'I'm going to help you get dressed, Rose. Is that okay?'

She looks at me with a frown. Her face is etched with deep wrinkles and she has white hairs on her chin. Her sharp blue eyes stare almost through me, and I wonder if she understands what I'm saying. I help her out of bed and into the chair and begin to change the sheets, wipe down the mattress and dry it, before putting new sheets on the bed and pulling them to the corners. I have been taught hospital corners – the practice of carefully folding the edges into a neat triangle so that the sheet does not ruffle up or cause pressure areas – and, despite being shown hundreds of times, I struggle with them, and my bed-making skills would not win any prizes.

Rose watches me, an ever-increasing frown splitting her forehead in two. She stands up suddenly. 'Do they not teach you young nurses anything in nursing school?' she says and, in one swift movement, she pulls the sheet out and performs the neatest and best hospital corner I've ever seen. I can feel my mouth drop open. It's as if she's suddenly alive, awake and alert. She was in a coma, of sorts, and then fully conscious.

It turns out that Rose was a nurse.

'Once a nurse, always a nurse,' the sister, Maggie, tells me. She is a square-shouldered woman with giant calf muscles, who smokes cigarettes despite being heavily pregnant. Times change. There is a hospital smoking room, where the staff and patients all mingle to smoke, which reminds me of a late-night jazz club, with thick yellow air and mustard walls that you could scrape layers of tar off with a knife. 'So we let her be a nurse.'

I'm not sure what she means, but I understand later, when I see Rose at the nurses' station rolling up bandages. The bandages we have are ready-rolled, so I can only assume that

Maggie has taken bandages out of the cellophane wrapping, unrolled them all and put them in a tray, before asking Rose to help. Whatever the logic, I can see at once that it is thera-peutic. Rose is alert and awake and is interacting with her environment and with others. She is convinced that she is my manager, and so when it's time for me to measure her blood pressure with a sphyg, I let her talk to me and correct my technique. 'Silly girl,' she says, as I place the stethoscope in the wrong place, unable to hear the pounding beat. 'Honestly, you have so much to learn about nursing.' She is not wrong.

I'm learning from the best nurses, though. Always. Today I am in the Cotswolds at a care home, talking to the nursing team who manage the residents' care. They show me to the nurses' station, which they've made into a post office, so that the residents with dementia might be 'encouraged to send letters and connect with the world'. Then there are the bath-rooms, which have been given a beach theme for one particular resident. 'She thought we were assaulting her, whenever we tried to help her bathe. Imagine how traumatic that must have been. So now we have a day at the beach and she enjoys it, says she loves "swimming in the sea".'

These nurses are innovative, making a huge difference to people's lives with their creative energy and ideas. As well as primary-care nursing, nursing in care-home settings is coor-dinated and preventative and seeks to maximise quality of life – rather than always focus on cure or length of life. 'I come to work,' one nurse in the care home tells me, 'and am able to make such a difference to families.' She flashes me a look. 'Or be with people when they die. Once, it was suggested that we take our residents out the back entrance after they die. But instead we all of us go through the front door, form a guard of honour – residents and staff alike. It's a comfort to all of us to know that respect is our priority.'

Rose does not live in a nursing home. Nor does she appear to be anywhere near close to death. I am astonished to discover that she lives at home, with no nursing input or carers. When Maggie tells me that Rose is cared for by her mother, I assume she is joking. But she is not. Florence, the mother, arrives mid-morning, carrying a tray of toad-in-the-hole that she has cooked 'for the nurses'. It turns out that she, too, was a nurse. She is now 104 years old and cares for Rose full-time and, aside from Rose's kidney infection, they apparently manage independently.

I have so many questions. I want to ask how on earth they cope with the practical challenges of life? How Florence stays so fit at 104 years old. How nursing was for them both, pre-NHS, through wars and life I can't even imagine. But I'm too taken aback to find out. All I can do is watch as they hug each other briskly, before Florence begins to help Rose roll up the bandages and sort syringes into different trays, depending on size. I look in their matching sharp blue eyes and imagine all they've seen. Maggie tells me that they've been on their own since diphtheria killed Florence's husband. He died, like so many others, before vaccines were widely available. Pre-NHS. The times they have lived through.

Rebecca is fourteen when I meet her on the general paediatric ward, where I'm working a night shift as a children's nurse. I'm glad to be here. Sandra says that A&E is already filling up with firework injuries, drunken teens and burns. It is Bonfire Night and I can see fireworks outside the window. It's a beautiful night and there's a star-filled clear sky, between bursts of colour. But Rebecca can't see. She has profound physical and learning disabilities, and has MRSA, so she needs to be nursed in a cubicle. A year ago she was fit and well, able bodied, academic and 'talked non-stop and was pretty wild'. There is a photo next to her bed of her and her boyfriend, Reece, the pair of them mischievous, pulling funny faces at the camera, holding ice-cream cones, with the sea in the background.

'Not my idea – she's too young.' Her stepdad, Philip, is a teacher. He talks about the pressures of teaching, and we compare notes with nursing: 'All public-sector jobs are under-valued and underpaid.' Rebecca's mum, Julia, is a full-time mother at home with Rebecca and two other children, who are now staying with their grandparents.

Philip sits on the plastic chair next to Rebecca's bed. He looks at the photo for a long time, then at his daughter. 'He's a lovely boy, Reece. Still visits her occasionally. But it's really hard for him, obviously.'

I am attaching a large bag of nutritional feed to a nasogastric tube that snakes down into Rebecca's nostril, then her throat, then her stomach. It is well taped to her face, but still, she keeps pulling it out accidentally. She will sooner or later get a gastrostomy PEG, to avoid the trauma of having a nasogastric tube and, particularly, having it reinserted so often. I remember in training when we put nasogastric tubes down each other. It probably isn't done now, but unpleasant as it was – causing us to cough and splutter and, in the case of my friend, vomit – I'm glad we did it. I never underestimate how uncomfortable it is for patients. The gastrostomy feeding tube has been discussed with Julia and Philip as a more permanent, less invasive way that Rebecca can get nutrition, but they are not yet ready to hear the truth that underlies that discussion. The words behind the medical language are simple, yet they are difficult to hear. The doctor says, 'A gastrostomy PEG stands for "percutaneous endoscopic gastrostomy" – it's a flexible feeding tube placed through the abdominal wall and into the stomach, and allows bypassing of the mouth and oesophagus in order that Rebecca receives adequate nutrition.' This can be translated to: 'Rebecca needs a permanent feeding tube because she will probably never eat or drink normally again.'

Rebecca contracted measles a year ago. Her parents had chosen not to vaccinate her. They understood that the research suggesting there was a link between the MMR (measles, mumps and rubella) vaccine and autism had been proven to be fake, and the doctor who published it had been struck off, but they were undeterred from their decision. Their health visitor spent many hours trying to listen and understand them; their school nurse attempted health promotion; and the primary-care nurse from the GP's surgery had many chats with the family about the importance of immunisation, the research about safety and the potential consequences of communicable diseases, for both Rebecca and others who might have poor immune systems. It is often the nurses who try to explain the importance of immunising children, for that individual child, and for other children too. 'Herd immunity' is a form of indirect protection against infectious diseases, meaning that if a percentage of the population receives vaccination, or develops antibodies, then epidemics of the disease are less likely. Everyone benefits from vaccination, but for the people most at risk – patients suffering from cancer, for example – it is literally lifesaving. A decision not to vaccinate a child puts other people's lives at risk: those with heart failure, the very young, the very old, those suffering from autoimmune conditions and those with cancer. Despite being told this and understanding it, the family chose not to immunise. In a world of 'fake news', it's hard to know who to trust, who to listen to. And sometimes we get it very wrong.

Rebecca developed significant irreparable and irreversible brain damage when she contracted complications after measles – one of the things that can happen. She cannot talk, sit, eat, laugh or smile. She has been left with a movement disorder that means she has constant jerks and spasms and moves continuously and involuntarily. Her entire body is tense. This will continue for the rest of her life. Other seemingly simple diseases of childhood can be equally life-altering, or even fatal. A baby with chickenpox whom I look after (his parents took him to a 'chickenpox party') dies, despite everyone's very best efforts. There have been increasing numbers of meningitis cases in recent years, as children who were not vaccinated are now old enough to attend music festivals and large gatherings and start sharing bodily fluids. These children can be left permanently deaf, without limbs and brain-damaged. Vaccination is still a choice. People can choose to manage their own risks. But when a population does not vaccinate, the risks to those who are immunosuppressed are significant. Those with cancer or any kind of immunodeficiency often do not have the luxury of choice.

'She was an artist,' Julia says. 'So brilliant at art. And pottery. She wanted to go to art school. She was a bit of a hellraiser, too.' She pauses. Rebecca has finally fallen asleep and her movements have subsided.

'Ah, the world always needs more hellraisers,' I say. I am going through Rebecca's drug chart, which is four pages long.

She is on all manner of medication: anti-seizure, pain relief, reflux medication, diuretics, anti-spasm drugs. I have to crush all the tablets and put them in her nasogastric tube, then flush them down with a lot of water to make sure they reach her stomach. I'm trying to concentrate and check the doses, but it's clear that Julia wants to talk.

We sit at a small sofa, and she tells me what she needs to. Rebecca was grounded; she had been out with Reece the day before and had come home two hours late. She disappeared to her bedroom and didn't emerge all day, and when Julia went in with toast and a cup of tea – to 'use the word "disappointed"' – Rebecca was complaining of a headache. She had a temperature and a sore throat, but nothing serious. The next day she was much the same and almost back to normal: cheeky, argumentative, moaning about being grounded during half-term. But the next day the rash started. It covered her head and neck first, then her whole body. She was laughing about it. 'We didn't think it was serious,' Julia says. 'It was only measles. But we sent the other two children to grannies.' She looks hollow. 'But then Rebecca started fitting. She started moving, and never really stopped.' She swallows so hard her entire neck moves. I put my arm loosely around her shoulder. It's all I can do.

Julia opens her handbag and takes out a small digital camera and a tissue. She switches the camera on and shows me the photos. Rebecca doing pottery. Rebecca on a waterslide.

On a horse. More pottery. More art. Watercolours and a series of birds. Rebecca laughing with friends. A shrine in stills.

I look at the photos of Rebecca doing pottery. 'I'm not into pottery, but my mum is,' I say. 'She loves art, too.' I think about my mum. She loves Japanese pottery. In Japan, broken pottery – like bowls or cups or vases – is often repaired with gold. It's called *Kintsugi*. And the flaws make the things even more beautiful than before. My mum only ever sees the gold in people. I spend my life trying to copy that. Kindness is learning the art of precious scars.

Julia looks over at Rebecca. Then she looks at me and dries her eyes with the tissue. 'This is my fault.'

And I try and see the gold in Julia, like my mum surely would. And be understanding, and forgiving, and compassionate. I try and switch off the voice inside me and listen instead to my mum's voice.

Rebecca contracted pneumonia and meningitis *and* encephalitis as a complication of measles. Complications of childhood diseases are rare, thankfully, but nurses have seen up close just how devastating they can be. German measles, or rubella, is an infection caused by the rubella virus, which can be prevented by the MMR vaccine. It is a common infection that, for most people, causes a short and not serious illness, and then complete recovery. But if rubella is contracted within the first twenty weeks of pregnancy, it can be dangerous, causing miscarriage, stillbirth and Congenital Rubella Syndrome.

An elderly man I care for in my very first pre-qualifying job was born with a patent ductus arteriosus (hole in the heart), severe learning disabilities, seizures and cataracts, and was later also diagnosed with diabetes, schizophrenia, autism and deafness, after his mum contracted rubella in pregnancy, back before the MMR vaccine existed. 'They call it "blueberry muffin syndrome". He had blue-reddish spots all over him and underneath his skin.' His mother is in her nineties and a wheelchair user herself. 'My husband told the doctor it was pretty offensive, but I liked it actually. That's why I call him "Blue" sometimes. My little Blue.' She ruffles the remaining hair on his almost-bald head. 'Blue.'

Congenital Rubella Syndrome is thankfully rare here, although it affects 100,000 babies around the world each year, but measles is now making a huge and terrifying comeback in the UK and internationally. It is one of the most highly infectious diseases, and more than 90 per cent of people will contract it, if they come into contact with it. Luckily, Reece was vaccinated, but who else did Rebecca have contact with, before showing symptoms? If a person with measles coughs in a room, and another unvaccinated person enters the room an hour or two later, they can contract the virus. Viruses outsmart us all the time; they live on paper, surfaces, hands. The World Health Organization recently reported that the measles epidemic has reached a thirteen-year high, with more than 500,000 cases reported from more than 180 countries in 2019. Meanwhile in America, where measles was supposedly eliminated in 2000, the Centers for Disease Control and Prevention report that there is now the largest measles outbreak for the last twenty-five years. In New York it led to a state of emergency and to a threat of fines for any resident who refused to vaccinate their children.

This kind of state intervention seemed extreme at the time. Of course everything has changed now. We live in a different world since COVID-19. How that world will take shape – how our lives will be lived – remains to be seen. But what is certain is that nothing will be the same.

Rebecca will live. But I've cared for patients who have died from such complications. And one thing I do know is this: nurses and doctors immunise their children.

Rebecca jolts awake to the sound of a rocket exploding outside, the screech and whoosh of fireworks and distant clapping and laughter. These sounds, which should delight any child, are making her anxious and jumpy. She makes a noise that is somewhere between a moan and a cry. Julia is shouting. Philip's head pops out from the curtain, calling me over.

It's the middle of the night. I hold a finger to my lips and whisper, 'Are you okay?'

Julia has covered her nose and mouth with her hand. She is giving Rebecca a change and a wash, and Rebecca is lying on her incontinence pad wearing just a pyjama top when I walk over. 'Look.' Julia pulls the pad a fraction, pointing to an area of rusty blood.

I stroke Rebecca's hair. 'Hey, Rebecca, this is Christie. I'm going to help Mum give you a wash.'

Rebecca's body jolts and spasms.

I whisper as I pull on an apron, and lean down to the bedside drawer to get some new pads. 'It looks like Rebecca is getting her period,' I say. And I stand up. Philip puts his arm around Julia, whose hand drops down. They look completely lost, both of them, as if they have woken up suddenly and don't know where they are.

'She was a terrible teenager,' Philip says. He is crying now, helpless.

Rebecca is thrashing around, grinding her teeth, her eyes rolling in different directions. She smells of sweat and an infection, pseudomonas, despite the wash we gave her two hours ago. Her body is on such high alert, and she's sweating so heavily, that I have to monitor her closely for fluid balance and any signs of dehydration. Her muscles are tense and wasting, her limbs skinny and at odd angles. I feel such sadness for her. I find it hard to look at the expression on her parents' faces. But I force myself. People say your life flashes before your eyes at the precise moment you die. But I see the flashes in their eyes. Their life then – how things were. How things will never be again. I busy myself making Rebecca comfortable.

Julia cannot speak at all. There are no words for this.

But Philip helps me roll Rebecca. 'I'd give anything to hear her slam a door again,' he says.

We are peak door-slamming age. Even so, now that my daughter is fifteen and my son is thirteen, not a day goes by when I don't remember the privilege it is to parent them. We are so lucky, I tell my children, and myself. Life is so precious. They have always been close, but are closer than ever now. I remember, early on, the anxiety that our social workers had – that I had – about adopting: how it might affect both the child joining the family and my existing birth child. But I don't know any siblings who are as close as my children. And they underestimated my daughter – who is, very much, the child of a nurse. Of course there are difficult days. Being a single parent isn't all easy. Being any parent isn't. But nursing has taught me so much. And over the years my patients and their relatives have taught me the biggest truth: the only thing that matters, in the end, is family. And families come in all shapes and sizes. Often we don't realise how lucky we are until something goes wrong, and then we realise how lucky we *were*.

There are days when I'm working and they're off to school, a flurry of activity and cleaning and organising, and rushing around and trying to get through a hundred emails and a never-ending to-do list on top of my full-time work, when I stop for a second. Nursing has gifted me the ability to be present and understand that these *are* the days. These every days – with all the stresses and strains of normal life – are the magical ones. There is no accident or emergency, or serious illness or birth, or death or violence; no significant life event, wedding or funeral or christening or graduation. Nursing gives magic to these days. The mundanity of human existence is where I find the most beauty; where I stop and absorb the significance of us – of nature, of humanity. It takes my breath away: how fragile, extraordinary and vulnerable, how full of hatred and love and obsession and complexity we all are – every single one of us.

I don't need to see the Northern Lights or a shooting star to feel my heart burst, to feel my most grateful, most alive, most human. I simply watch my children eating their breakfast. They catch me watching them sometimes: studying their faces, their expressions, staring at them, unblinking. 'You're so weird, Mum,' they tell me, laughing. But I can't stop. I don't want to blink. Because, in a flash, it will be over.

12

Nurses' Hands

December is a time of worry in hospitals. It is always too busy and every year it gets busier. The *Help Us Help You* posters, trying to send people away, start going up:

IF YOU HAVE CHEST PAIN, call 999.
IF YOU HAVE FLU, go to your GP.
IF YOU HAVE MILD INJURIES OR INFECTIONS, go to your pharmacy.

There are planning and contingency meetings, and 'worst-case scenario' is a term that starts to float around boardrooms. Critical-incident policies are reviewed in preparation for terrorist attacks or biological warfare, or ebola or coronavirus, although we have no real idea what is to come. We can't even begin to imagine. We spend days fitting staff with masks, in the event of bird flu or SARS, and planning ward-quarantine areas; and we stock up on obscure antiviral drugs that are not proven to be effective, but are all we have. There are so many meetings. They almost always comprise the same people discussing the same things as the week before, and nobody has actioned anything. 'It's like Groundhog Day,' a nurse manager tells me. 'Same old shit, different day.'

Flu season does come yearly, though, and the most worrying part is the number of staff who may need two weeks off. Making all NHS staff have a flu jab is not done to protect them from the illness, but to protect the organisation from their sick days. December moves on. Old wards are identified that can be used for overflow, when the inevitable happens. There's a pause before things get busier and busier – and I've always found that pause to be a time when I've reflected most on my own actions and experiences. The weight of my choices. Life happens at such speed that perhaps it is in these quiet moments, when things are calm, that our internal life is richest. When we examine who we really are and what we are made of. And when we begin to question our humanity, our vulnerability and even our morality.

As frontline staff, we live in spaces where sometimes there is no right or wrong, only the in-between. We are always questioning our actions: whether they were enough, or even right. 'Do No Harm' is not always possible, despite our best efforts. Often medicine and nursing are choices between bad or worse, not good or better. The only way I can cope with this is to think always of compassion. To ask myself difficult questions, and keep the patient and their family at the heart of all things. To treat them as if they were my own loved ones. I always assumed nursing was about saving lives. That patients want that at all costs, or, at least, families do. I was wrong. Compassion is the thing that matters most to patients and their families. Dignity, respect and compassionate care.

Henry is the most beautiful baby I've ever seen. I'm allocated to care for him, in cubicle five, for a long day of twelve and a half hours; and I have four such shifts in succession, so I will probably spend all that time next to him, getting to know his family in an intense and emotional way. Henry is eighteen months old and has been admitted to hospital with encephalitis, a serious virus that attacks the brain. He's suffered seizure after seizure for six days, each one longer than the last, each more difficult to manage with medication, until one seizure doesn't stop at all. Henry's tiny body arches backwards, his fists clench and his eyes roll so far back that I can only see the whites. His head flicks rhythmically to the right every second. His feet extend in a ballet pose.

'Where is he?' his mum, Shirley, asks loudly. 'Where's my baby? He doesn't look real. It's like a horror film.'

And Henry does look possessed. A zombie-horror version of a baby. Twisted, fighting an unseen enemy.

We have to put him into a medical thiapentonal coma, to sedate and medically paralyse him until the jerking, twisting and jolting stop. While the doctors are discussing burst suppression and pharmacological neuroprotection, and are analysing complex treatment plans, I hold Shirley's hand. With her other hand she strokes Henry's head.

'No more suffering,' she whispers. 'Please, no more suffering.'

Neurological conditions are my main interest at work, and I'm currently writing a policy for the management of neurological emergencies, obsessed with research into the most valuable treatment of herniation. Treatments of all kinds in hospital are seasonal and fall in and out of fashion – just like hospital structure itself. We see PICUs become regional, then centralised, then regional again, the new managers reinventing the wheel every few years. And the senior nurses have seen it all before; 'full circle' is a term we know all too well.

'We're going back to the way we did it twenty years ago, and in ten years we'll revert back again,' Tracy, one of the most experienced PICU nurses, tells me, 'and what a bloody waste of time and money that is. If only they asked the nurses.' Indeed, policy-making nurses are few and far between, and even when hospitals are built, it's a fight to get nurses consulted. She tells me about a ward she worked on which was shiny and new and built with a glass exterior that had to be redesigned when the ward had a tropical climate all year round, despite the air conditioning. 'Any nurse would have told the architect that extreme heat and bacteria are not a good mix.' And Tracy rushes off, hurriedly eating a piece of toast. She is always rushing, even though today it is fairly calm and quiet.

The winter cold snap and the year's busiest time are nearly upon us. But before the storm comes the calm: there is time for reflection and for planning. Even if we're not aware of it, we are in tune with nature. Like hospitals, our own bodies can be calm before the storm. When people are about to die, they often have a lucid period when everything is quiet and still. Relatives will comment that their loved one seems to have perked up and looks better. And the nurses know this is an indication that death is imminent; they are in the process of a strange meditation, the stripping back of their lives. Just as midwives know the full moon will bring babies, so nurses understand that the final days and hours before death are when people often seem at their most peaceful.

It is a few weeks later and Henry is still now. He is in multi-organ failure and has irrecoverable brain damage. 'The doctors have explained that he will never wake up,' Shirley tells me. 'The machines are just prolonging his death.' Medical ethics – autonomy, beneficence and non-maleficence, justice – are as important to critical care as medication and technology. Perhaps more so. With the wishes and consent of Henry's family at the heart of the conversation about his care, it has been decided by the consultant and the multi-disciplinary team that Henry's treatment will be withdrawn. Shirley tells me she wants Henry to have a natural death. Henry will be taken off the ventilator today, and have his breathing tube taken out. Shirley looks at the machines. 'The only thing keeping him alive for now is this breathing machine. They've stopped the dialysis, and the heart drugs.' She picks up his hand, folds his tiny fingers around hers. 'I don't want him to die like this. Not on machines. I will not have my son suffer any more.'

We have no way of saving Henry's life, but allowing him a pain-free and dignified death is so important, and the memories of that will last a lifetime for his family. Every detail matters. I make sure the crash trolley is not too near. I tell the team under no circumstances to put out a crash call for the baby in bed five. The last thing I need is a room filled with a crash team, or an eager member of staff who doesn't know the circumstances trying to resuscitate him. I make sure the DNACPR documentation is nearby and all correct. I pick the quietest time when the other parents of children have gone for some lunch. We don't know what will happen. Henry might breathe a while, or he might not. I plan to give him high-flow oxygen to make things easier for him, and he is already on a morphine infusion for pain relief. He will be comfortable whatever happens. I prepare as much as I can. But I still don't feel prepared. Something is pulling at my insides, scratching me. There's a taste of dust in my mouth; a dull ache at the back of my head. I feel wrong, somehow, like I've forgotten something really important.

We set a time: 1 p.m. And all I can think of all day is what I need to do. All the details which will matter so much. Being a nurse is so often about saving lives. But today being a nurse is about allowing death. The death of a child. A baby. Allowing a natural death seems at odds with nature.

I am caring for Henry in a side-room. I dim the lights, half-close the blinds, put out a jug of fresh water and some cups. I check and double-check that I have enough suction catheters and the right-sized oxygen mask. I know that Henry will not be attached to a mechanical ventilator, but there are still things I can do for him, withdrawal of treatment is not withdrawal of care: oxygen, suction, fluids, medication. I change the bedside chairs for the comfiest I can find, and choose pillows with new pillowcases to put on them. I even examine the pillowcases to make sure they have no tiny tears or smudges. I find a box of tissues.

The consultant pops in on me. 'Are you sure you're okay to do this?'

It is usually the doctors here who remove endotracheal tubes in this kind of scenario. But the parents want me to do it. Shirley asked me. So of course I said yes, although I feel sick and unsure, and I'm shaking. I think of my medical colleagues who make big decisions that have life-lasting consequences. The weight of consultant-led decisions that doctors must bear.

'I'll be fine,' I say, certain that I will. I'm not causing this child to die. The encephalitis has done that job. I am removing the technology that is preventing a natural death – that's all. But I don't feel fine, suddenly. And death is never natural for a child. It's against the order of everything. It is never right for a child – a baby – to die. Not in any circumstance. But keeping patients barely alive at all costs with technology, and prolonging suffering, is not right, either.

I am as ready as I'll ever be, with Shirley sitting down on the chair, a pillow plumped over her forearm, and Henry lying on top; Andrea, her partner, is on the chair next to her. But I find that my throat is burning from holding in tears and my hands are clammy. My skin goosebumps with fear.

Henry is not conscious, yet he seems to look at me with his completely still and perfectly green eyes. I slowly unwind the plaster that is holding down the tube in his nose – the tube attached to the breathing machine that is keeping him alive. I've seen this done many times. A baby or a child will not suddenly struggle to breathe. He should be comfortable. It is likely that gradually the carbon dioxide in Henry's body will rise, and he'll eventually breathe less and less and will die peacefully and naturally. But I don't know that for sure. We never really know anything for sure.

I have turned off all the monitors. We don't need to see them. I gently take the tube out and watch Shirley's face, then Henry's. Henry's body takes a deep, reflexive breath. His eyes are half-open, but he is comatose. He is far away. I count slowly backwards from 100 in my head. We are all counting backwards. My many years of nursing give me the numbers. Henry reaches seven.

Shirley kisses his head, presses her cheek to his. 'No more suffering,' she says. 'No more suffering.'

When COVID-19 arrives, its impact is devastating and we are yet to see all the changes and damage it will cause. One area it has already altered drastically is nursing. Nurses in critical care are used to delivering one-to-one care to the sickest patients on life-support machines, ventilators and strong heart drugs, kidney dialysis machines – taking over from a person's body when they are in multi-organ failure. We are told that within weeks the UK will reach a peak but that critical-care capacity has been increased in order to deal with it. But you can't simply increase critical-care capacity overnight without consequence. We have been working over capacity for years already. We are afraid, none more so than critical care nurses, who understand that the importance and skill and expertise of their job can't be learned overnight. Critical care is more than just ventilators, it's rigorously trained specialist nurses. We are worried about the level of quality and safety in critical care during this pandemic, and equally worried about rehab and long-term care for patients afterwards.

I can't imagine what COVID-19 will do to the nurses: what deeds they will have to perform, what scars they will have to bear. The horror of what is to come is always informed by what has passed and, as nurses, we have all cared for people who have died who should not have died. But people dying in greater numbers because they are elderly and happen to live in care homes, or because they are black or from Bangladeshi, Indian or Pakistani ethnicities, or because they are healthcare workers who may not have had the appropriate PPE. These thoughts are hard to even contemplate. We have all experienced those days that we will never forget, but maybe all days over the coming months will be worse than the previous day. Watching someone die before their time and knowing that they might have lived is indescribable. Watching people die due to inequality and discrimination is completely unbearable. We all need to hold onto this anger, fight this horrific injustice. Meanwhile, during this time of COVID-19, nurses and health and social care workers will be there for everyone, regardless. Critical care nurses, and all nurses, will be there, even when relatives cannot be. Holding the hand of a loved one, when that is all they can offer. Being family, when family are not there.

It will be nurses holding the hand of every person in hospital who dies from this virus. And nurses holding the hand of every person in hospital who dies from everything else at this time. Families everywhere say that's the worst thing: knowing their loved one was alone during their final, darkest hours. But nobody will ever be alone while there are nurses. Nurses are there, always. They always have been, and they always will be. And no matter who we are, or how we've lived, or what choices we've made, nurses – the good ones – care for their patients as unconditionally as if they are family. It seems a simple task in nursing. But what an honour that is: to hold the hand of a person when they are most alone, most frightened and most human. To be a nurse.

My son is now thirteen and he loves basketball. I think of all the patients I've ever looked after. I think of Jason with his basketball. Of India's pain. Of Danny and Michael. I think of my patients over the years. Some people are not easy to care for – most people. Patients aren't always grateful, and they don't always want help. But morality is complex and is not for individuals to decide upon. I watch my son and think of what might have been, what might be to come. And I know that all I can do is cherish every moment, every minute.

I think of the other families like Henry's who aren't lucky enough to watch their child grow up. I think of my son's birth mother's pain. I watch my son throw the ball through the net a million times and every time turn to the kitchen window to check that I'm watching and saw the hoop. I put my thumbs up each time. Eventually he comes in, hungry as ever, and I make him a sandwich and we sit and talk. We always talk about everything. But during the holidays we talk more. It is Christmas Day tomorrow and I wonder why he doesn't seem excited. And then he asks me about his birth family.

And I remember that for some children, for some adults, and for some families, the big significant days are the hardest days of all. He hardly ever mentions adoption. But today he wants to.

'Do you think my birth family are into basketball?' He looks out of the window, avoiding my eyes. He worries about my pain, about her pain – about everyone. 'Because I'm pretty obsessed.'

I'm ready for this. I've been saving these gifts for a long time. These hidden-away Christmas presents are the most important of all. He looks at me, checks he hasn't hurt me. 'I'm not sure,' I say. 'When you write to them next, why not ask them.'

He writes to his birth family twice a year – something called 'letterbox contact'. Contact between adopted children and their birth families is encouraged and can vary from face-to-face contact in specialist contact centres, usually for older children, to yearly or twice-yearly letterbox contact. Every January and August we send a letter and photos to a contact centre, which then passes them on, and vice versa. These letters are so important to my son. And when I mention writing, I worry there's a sadness deep inside him. It's difficult to reach, but I will always try. I begin to tell him what I know. What I promised. What you can't read from reports or learn from social workers.

In the light, your birth mum's eyes change colour from brown to hazelnut and they are flecked with gold, just like yours.

You laugh so much like her, and she snorts, too, when she laughs a lot.

You have the same long fingers.

She crosses her legs exactly like you do.

She is so beautiful, just as you are.

'Err, handsome,' he replies. He looks at his fingers and smiles. Then he picks up my hand and presses our fingers together, palm to palm. 'Your fingers are ridiculously short,' he says.

'When you were little, you always used to call them sausage fingers,' I say, and somehow we laugh. And I keep hold of his hand, warm and long-fingered.

I watch his face, mesmerised, and I realise something important. I get to hold his hand for always – wherever life takes us. What a privilege that is. It's not always right. And it's never perfect. Adoption means a child will never belong to you completely. Not really. But that doesn't matter at all, because I belong to him for ever.

Afterword

I am walking once more across the bridge. Behind me, the Houses of Parliament are empty. In front of me, the hospital is full of people seriously ill and dying. And there are no families. No relatives. The bridge is empty of cars and people, even rough sleepers. I wonder where they have gone. Perhaps they have died. I close my eyes for the briefest of seconds and see the parish nurse, Rachel, herself a single mother like me, wandering the streets at night – on her days off – to look for homeless people she might help, or give soup to; a blanket, first aid, medical care. I picture her sitting down next to someone broken, alone and vulnerable, someone difficult and angry and maybe even violent. I see her reaching out, even then, for that person's hand. When I open my eyes I look at the water, no longer as polluted, changing colours once more, from grey and green to blue, the way my dad's eyes changed colour depending on the light – or his mood, he insisted.

This bridge has seen some things. The terrorist attack in March 2017, when nurses and doctors saved as many lives as they could, indiscriminately. Teams of nurses and doctors and healthcare workers risking stress, PTSD, burnout, infection, terrorism.

I think of Eamonn talking about teamwork. I remember the photo on his desk of the beautiful young family who needs him. I imagine them now, waving him off to spend months trying to set up a hospital, knowing that there is a chance he will come home different, haunted. We all will, wherever we work. I think of his wife missing him so much, but of the smile she will no doubt put on her face. Of her bravery, too. The grit of all the families of nurses.

Looking out at the river, I hear the voice of Jess from the Queen's Nursing Institute Scotland. Jess's voice is the one that gives me most strength. It makes me laugh, even when it's not really funny. There are pauses in her humour right now; chinks of darkness making it through even her strength. Her husband has cancer. He is going for a big operation tomorrow while she remains working as a frontline nurse in the police cells. At best, they might have to be apart at this, the worst time of their lives. I ask her if they would consider postponing the operation, as the risk of him catching COVID-19 is so high. She says they have thought about it. But she knows, as I do, that this thing could go on for a year. Years even. Healthcare may never catch up or recover. She also knows, as I do, that a cancer year is a very long time. While this virus is spreading across our world, cancer is spreading across hers. I know how that feels. 'We're going for it,' she says. Her voice is strong once more, for her husband, and for herself. 'Because I quite like him.'

I walk slowly at first, thinking some more, trying to learn from these women and men. I am so worried for my mum, on her own on the Isle of Man. And for my nan, shielding and in her nineties. These incredible women who raised me – and made me – taught me the language of kindness. I hate thinking of them alone. These times are so lonely for so many of us. But loneliness is no longer the disease of the elderly. I stop for a moment and text my children. They have grown up overnight. I am a single parent and my fifteen-year-old daughter, instead of going out to parties and falling in love for the first time, and taking risks and doing all the things fifteen-year-olds should be doing, is offering to stay on top of her home schooling and help keep a close eye on her younger brother, so that I can work long days in nursing. She is planning to cook, so that there is a meal waiting when I get home from work. I tell her she doesn't need to do that, because her adult sister – her dad's eldest – has offered to stay to help while I work, but she is already writing a menu. Pesto pasta features heavily. My ex and his partner – also an intensive-care consultant – offer to help, having the children between us, depending on who is working; or, as we predict, who is inevitably sick at some stage. Family is a funny thing. Blended, mixed up, complex and yet, in that mixture, during these times, it is also very clear.

'I feel bad about not focusing on you. I feel like we ought to be together during this time. I should put you first,' I say at home.

'Will you help people?' my daughter asks. I nod and tell them I'm rusty but that, with training and support, I'll help the nurses, and the patients and their families. I'm planning to help for the first peak though I have no idea how long that peak will last. 'Do it,' she says.

And my son nods and puts on his determined expression. 'You must.'

People are talking a lot about bravery during these times. But I don't feel at all brave. I feel fear. And guilt. I spend an afternoon watching my son play basketball in the garden. I am crying. How could I risk getting sick? I feel selfish. And then he looks up at the window, too far away to see my tears, and waves, then spins the basketball on his finger and does some sort of silly dance move. And my daughter comes into my bedroom, carrying a cup of tea. She puts the tea down and grins. 'We'll be fine, you know,' she says. She looks down at her brother. 'He'll be fine.' She flicks her head back at me – defiant as ever. And strong. 'We want you to do this. Besides, the rest of the time, when you're not at work you'll be home, annoying us like always.'

And I stand back and look at her grinning, this daughter of mine, remembering her newly born, curled up in a hedgehog ball. How astonishing she has turned out to be. I may not be feeling brave, but my children are. It is always from them that I find the courage to care.

Still, I feel pain. I feel such pain for the patients who will lose their lives, and the relatives who won't be there to hold their hands. I think of the nurses and doctors and health and social care workers who will risk their lives – even before I know about the issues across the country with limited PPE supplies – and may suffer moral injury and mental illness as a result of their jobs. These ordinary women and men living in extraordinary times, simply getting on with it. I am frightened. But a pull overrides everything else and sits in my chest, filling a hole that I never knew existed. I can taste it in my mouth and feel it on my skin.

I put my phone away and take a last, long look at the water. This river that swallows all stories. This huge story we are living through. My story. And yours. I start walking, slowly at first. But despite everything, my nurse's feet walk quicker, and I'm almost running. Running towards the hospital and, at first, I hear nothing but silence, the streets and roads empty of cars and humans. But as I run, I hear the sound of alarms, and shouting from the wards ahead, and there's an ambulance siren, and somewhere in the distance I hear a baby crying. I look up and see my mum, and somehow she is right there with me, and I know for the first time what that means; and I understand that whatever happens, whenever my daughter and my son look up, I will always be there. Always.

I run now, not because I'm in a rush, but because I can't stop. And I hear my heartbeat in my head and my shoes on the bridge; and I hear my dad: *It's amazing what you can do, with extra time*; and I hear the voice of my son's birth mother too; and I hear my nan asking Dorothy for a Marks and Spencer jumper, the cerise one; and Mum telling me it will all be okay; and my brother saying he invented Ibiza; and my children laughing together, their laughter syrupy, thicker than blood. And I think of the nurses I have worked with, these expert and compassionate people, and what they have taught me: Rachel and kindness, Eamonn and teamwork, Jess and resilience. I get to stand next to them, for a while at least, and my head spins with everything before and everything after. I wasn't a born nurse. But this pull of my feet and my heart and my head is older and deeper and stronger than I can describe in language. Maybe I got it wrong. Maybe we all got it wrong. Perhaps, after all, for me at least, this is a calling.

I slow down at the entrance and walk in, catching my breath. Hospitals have always been a sanctuary throughout history. Now is no different. But I always assumed they were a sanctuary for patients. I was wrong. I've been wrong about so many things. When life gives me the greatest challenges, it is in nursing that I find the most answers, the most comfort, the most lessons. Nurses remind me of who we human beings

are, and who we are meant to be. It is nurses who make me
want to be a better person.

My colleague, Sandra, is waiting for me at the entrance,
wearing scrubs and carrying a spare pair for me to change
into. We haven't seen each other for a few years, but there is
no time for small talk. She hands the scrubs over and nods.
'Welcome home.'

Acknowledgements

I want to thank my children, who encouraged me to tell parts of their story in the hope it helps other families affected by adoption. Parenting you is the greatest privilege of my life.

This book, as ever, is for nurses. It would not have been possible without the passionate work of everyone at my literary agency, C&W, and my publishers, Chatto & Windus and Vintage. Thank you to them, and to all individuals and communities everywhere who have supported keyworkers in many different ways.

To those hundreds of nurses and patients and family members who have shared with me their time and expertise, I am indebted to you. Many of you have asked me to not name you personally, and with that in mind I'll avoid listing thanks to individuals. You absolutely know who you are. I am so grateful for all you do. We all are.

Thank you:

Nurses.

And porters; midwives; healthcare assistants; doctors; allied health professionals; pharmacists; radiographers; speech and language therapists; dietitians; mortuary staff; operating department practitioners; health and social care managers; research teams; academics; scientists; lab technicians; refuse collectors; psychologists; counsellors; midwifery support workers; cleaners; firefighters; chefs; kitchen staff; phlebotomists; food-bank staff; audiologists; paramedics; ambulance drivers; physiotherapists; play therapists; family support and bereavement staff; chaplains; cardiac technicians; hospice staff; charity workers; taxi drivers; biomedical scientists; volunteers; security guards; teachers; teaching assistants; dental nurses; all at Royal Mail; police officers; delivery drivers; supermarket workers; bus, train, tram, Underground staff; call handlers; dentists; social workers; carers.

The RCN Foundation is committed to caring for the nurses who care for all of us. Throughout the COVID-19 pandemic, the Foundation has been providing emergency funding and psychological support to frontline staff. The RCN Foundation safeguards nurses, midwives and healthcare assistants facing hardship by providing advice and financial help to those in crisis. They invest in the future of nursing by funding learning and development. And they promote vital nurse-led research. I am proud to act as their patron.

To donate to the RCN Foundation, visit their website: https://rcnfoundation.rcn.org.uk/donate